6-23-78

THE
HOUSE & GARDEN
BOOK OF
TOTAL HEALTH

—THE—
HOUSE & GARDEN
—BOOK OF—
TOTAL HEALTH

Book planned by
Mary Jane Pool
Editor-in-Chief, *House & Garden*

Edited by
Caroline Seebohm
Senior Writer

G. P. Putnam's Sons • New York

All illustrations appearing in this book are the work of Durell Godfrey and Susan Dade and have been reprinted from past issues of *House & Garden Magazine*. The photographs on pages 370-372 are the work of Christian Reinhardt.
Acknowledgments for recipes reprinted in this book:
The recipe for Bran Muffins from *The Joy of Cooking* by Irma S. Rombauer and Marion R. Becker is reprinted by kind permission of Bobbs-Merrill Company, Inc.
The recipes for Scalloped Cabbage with Nutmeg Sauce by Mrs. Joe Hume Gardner, for Broccoli Mold by Mrs. William W. Magruder, and for Buttermilk Dressing by Mrs. John M. Young are all reprinted by kind permission of the authors from *The 1977 Stratford Hall Cookbook*.
The recipe for Lacy Oatmeal Cookies from *Private Collection: A Culinary Treasure* is reprinted by kind permission of the Private Art Collections Women's Committee of the Walters Art Gallery.
The recipes for Spinach Casserole, Potato Latkes, Easy Cheese Soufflé, and Wheat-Soy Waffles from *Diet for a Small Planet* by Frances Moore Lappé are reprinted by kind permission of Raines & Raines.
The recipe for Rice Bread from *Ricecraft* by Margaret Gin is reprinted by kind permission of Random House, Inc.

SBN: 399-12154-4

Library of Congress Cataloging in Publication Data

Main entry under title:

The House & garden book of total health.

A selection of articles from House & garden.
Includes index.
1. Health—Addresses, essays, lectures.
I. Pool, Mary Jane.   II. Seebolm, Caroline.
III. House & garden.   IV. Title: Book of total health
RA776.H825   613   78-5048

PRINTED IN THE UNITED STATES OF AMERICA

CONTENTS

7017488

from Corinne Caduff of Saks Fifth Avenue and massage step-by-step from Vicki Schick of the Profile Health Spa, New York. Interviews by Paula Rice Jackson.

PART TWO—NUTRITION AND FUEL FOR A HEALTHY BODY

reducing food, menus, and recipes. Interview by Jane Ellis. *3. Rancho La Puerta*—Deborah Mazzanti's other resort, with menus and recipes. Interview by Jane Ellis. *4. The Greenhouse Spa*—recipes and health tips from Helen Corbitt. Interview by Jane Ellis. *5. Eugénie-les-Bains*—Michel Guérard explains his famous *cuisine minceur* philosophy and recipes. Interview by Naomi Barry.

Dr. Willibald Nagler; skating from Dr. Tenley E. Albright; cross-country skiing from Dr. John L. Marshall; exercises for total fitness from Dr. Laurence E. Morehouse. Interviews by Caroline Seeboyhm.

ABOUT THE EXPERTS

DR. TENLEY E. ALBRIGHT   ° Skating °   Chapter 34

Dr. Albright is General Surgeon at the Sports Medicine Resource, Woburn, Massachusetts, and a member of the President's Council on Physical Fitness and Health. She won the 1956 Olympic Gold Medal for figure skating

DR. GREGORY BATESON   ° Psychology °   Chapter 42

Dr. Bateson is an anthropologist, psychologist, and author. He currently teaches anthropology, cybernetics, and genetics at Kresge College, University of California at Santa Cruz. Probably the best-known of his books is *Steps to an Ecology of Mind* (Ballantine).

DR. HERBERT BENSON   ° Psychology °   Chapter 46

Dr. Benson is Professor of Cardiology at Harvard Medical School, and Director, Hypertension Section, Beth Israel Hospital, Boston. His research into relaxation led him to write the book, *The Relaxation Response* (Morrow).

DR. ROBERT A. BERGER   ° Hair °   Chapter 11

Dr. Berger is Assistant Attending Dermatologist, Mount Sinai Hospital, and Assistant Clinical Professor, Mount Sinai School of Medicine, Department of Dermatology, in New York City.

DR. A. A. BRIDGER   ° Psychology °   Chapter 43

Dr. Bridger teaches at Columbia University, New York, and

is in private practice. He is particularly interested in the use of hypnosis for overweight patients and those who want to give up smoking.

DR. JORGE BUXTON   ° Eyes °   Chapter   8

Dr. Buxton is a surgeon and Director of the Corneal Clinic, New York Eye and Ear Infirmary. He is also Clinical Professor of Ophthalmology, College of Medicine, New Jersey Medical School. He specializes in corneal surgery.

DR. EDWARD COLT   ° Running °   Chapter   36

Dr. Colt is an endocrinologist at St. Luke's Hospital, New York. He is also physician for the New York Marathon, participant in metabolic studies projects on runners, and a runner himself.

DR. DENTON COOLEY   ° Heart °   Chapter   1

Dr. Cooley is Surgeon-in-Chief, Texas Heart Institute, and Surgical Consultant to St. Luke's Episcopal and Texas Children's Hospitals, Houston, Texas. His pioneering work in heart surgery has won him numerous awards from all over the world. He implanted the first artificial heart in 1967.

DR. WILLIAM C. COOPER   ° Eyes °   Chapter   8

Dr. Cooper is Associate Clinical Professor of Ophthalmology, Columbia Presbyterian Hospital, and Diplomate of the American Board of Ophthalmology. He specializes in orbit and reconstructive surgery.

HELEN CORBITT   ° Weight Control °   Chapters 30, 33

Helen Corbitt is food consultant to the Greenhouse Spa, Dallas, Texas, and a nutrition expert. She is author of *Helen*

Corbitt Cooks for Looks and *Helen Corbitt Entertains* (Houghton Mifflin).

MARJORIE CRAIG   ° Hands °   Chapter   10

Marjorie Craig, Director of Exercise at Elizabeth Arden, was trained in physiotherapy at the Neurological Institute at Columbia Presbyterian Medical Center in New York City.

DR. JOEL R. DAVITZ   ° Psychology °   Chapter   43

Dr. Davitz is Professor of Psychology, Teacher's College, Columbia University. He is also coauthor with his wife, Lois Leiderman Davitz, of *Making it From 40 to 50* (Random House).

DR. RENE DUBOS   ° Psychology °   Chapter   47

Dr. Dubos is a microbiologist, environmentalist, pathologist, and Professor Emeritus of Environmental Biomedicine at Rockefeller University, New York. He is the author of many books including the Pulitzer Prize-winning *So Human an Animal.*

DR. RICHARD G. EATON   ° Hands °   Chapter   10

Dr. Eaton runs the Hand Service, Department of Surgery, Roosevelt Hospital, New York. Dr. Eaton is also Associate Clinical Professor of Surgery at Columbia College of Physicians and Surgeons, New York.

DR. BERNARD E. FINNESON ° Backs °   Chapter   3

Dr. Finneson is Chief of Neurosurgery, Director of the Low Back Pain Clinic of the Crozer-Chester Medical Center, Chester, Pennsylvania, and Associate Professor of Neurological Surgery, Hahnemann Medical College, Philadelphia, Pennsylvania. He is also coauthor, with Arthur S. Freese, of *The New Approach to Low Back Pain* (Berkley & Windhover).

DR. DALE G. FRIEND ° Weight Control °   Chapter 31

Dr. Friend is Associate Clinical Professor of Medicine Emeritus, Harvard Medical School, and in private practice. He is a specialist in the field of drugs.

DR. ERICH FROMM   ° Psychology °   Chapter 41

Dr. Fromm is a world-famous psychoanalyst and author. He was formerly Professor of Psychoanalysis at Bennington College, Yale, Michigan State, and New York Universities. He is author of many books, including the *Revolution of Hope* and *The Art of Loving.* His most recent book is *To Have Or To Be* (Harper & Row).

DR. S. EVANS GANZ   ° Eyes °   Chapter   6

Dr. Ganz is Attending Surgeon, Manhattan Eye, Ear and Throat Hospital in New York City. Dr. Ganz is also Diplomate of the American Board of Otolaryngology.

DR. NATHANIEL GOULD   ° Feet °   Chapter   5

Dr. Gould is former Chief Orthopedic Surgeon at Brockton Hospital, Brockton Massachusetts. He is a founder of the American Orthopedic Foot Society.

DR. BERNARD GREEN   ° Psychology °   Chapter 44

Dr. Green is a New York psychotherapist, and founder of the International Awareness Center. Dr. Green is also a Fellow of the American Society for Psychical Research, and lecturer on psychotherapeutic techniques.

DR. MARCI GREENWOOD Weight Control ° Chapter 31

Dr. Greenwood is Assistant Professor of Human Genetics and Development, Institute of Human Nutrition, Columbia University, New York.

MICHEL GUERARD   ° Weight Control °   Chapter 30

Michel Guérard runs the famous health spa at Eugénie-les-Bains, in Les Landes, southwest France, where he practices the principles of *cuisine minceur.*

DR. WILLIAM G. HAMILTON   ° Bones °   Chapter 4

Dr. Hamilton is Orthopedic Surgeon, Roosevelt Hospital, New York, and Instructor in Orthopedics, Columbia University College of Physicians and Surgeons. He is also Orthopedist for the New York City Ballet, and Fellow of the American College of Surgeons.

DR. ERNEST HARTMANN   ° Sleep °   Chapter 39

Dr. Hartmann, a sleep expert, is Director of the Sleep and Dream Laboratory, Boston State Hospital, and Professor of Psychiatry, Tufts University School of Medicine.

DR. PETER HERMAN   ° Psychology °   Chapter 45

Dr. Herman is Assistant Professor of Psychology, University of Toronto. He specializes in research into the phenomenon of self-control in such areas as weight control.

DR. BERNARD JACOBS   ° Necks °   Chapter 6

Dr. Jacobs is Clinical Professor of Orthopedic Surgery,

Cornell University. Dr. Jacobs is also head of the Neck Clinic, New York's Hospital for Special Surgery.

DR. ANNA KARA   ° Skin °   Chapter   40

Dr. Kara is the Director, Physical Medicine and Rehabilitation Department, St. Clare's Hospital, Denville, New Jersey, and Assistant Clinical Professor in Medicine (Physical), Cornell University Medical College.

DR. ALBERT A. KATTUS   ° HEART °   Chapter   35

Dr. Kattus is a cardiologist and Professor of Medicine (Cardiology) at the University of California, Los Angeles. He is also former Chairman of the Exercise Committee, American Heart Association.

DR. ALBERT M. KLIGMAN   ° Skin °   Chapter   7

Dr. Kligman is Professor of Dermatology, University of Pennsylvania School of Medicine. He is also President of the Society for Investigative Dermatology, and publishes over a dozen professional papers a year.

LARRY LORENCE   ° Exercise °   Chapter   40

Mr. Lorence is an exercise expert and Director of Gala Fitness in New York. He has also appeared on television shows across the country demonstrating his exercise techniques.

DR. IRWIN D. MANDEL   ° Teeth °   Chapter   9

Dr. Mandel is Professor of Dentistry, and Director of the Division of Preventive Dentistry at Columbia University School of Dental and Oral Surgery.

DR. JOHN L. MARSHALL   ° Sports °   Chapters 4, 5, 34

Dr. Marshall is Director of Sports Medicine, New York's Hospital for Special Surgery, and Orthopedic Consultant to the New York School system. He is also orthopedist for the U.S. Ski Team, and a keen skier himself.

DEBORAH MAZZANTI ° Weight Control °   Chapter 30

Deborah Mazzanti is founder of the Golden Door health spa in Escondido, California, and Rancho La Puerto in Tecate, Mexico. She is a member of the President's Council on Physical Fitness and Health, and author of *Secrets of the Golden Door* (Morrow).

DR. JOSEPH MENDELS   ° Sleep °   Chapter 39

Dr. Mendels is Director of the Depression Clinic, Hospital of the University of Pennsylvania, and Professor of Psychiatry, University of Pennsylvania. Dr. Mendels is also Chief, Affective Diseases Research Unit, Veterans Administration Hospital, Philadelphia, Pennsylvania.

DR. LAURENCE E. MOREHOUSE ° Fitness ° Chapters 34, 38

Dr. Morehouse is founding Director of the Human Performance Laboratory, University of California, Los Angeles. He was Fitness Consultant to the NASA Space Program, and is the author of *Total Fitness in 30 Minutes a Week* and *Maximum Performance* (Simon & Schuster).

DR. WILLIBALD NAGLER   ° Joints °   Chapters 5, 34

Dr. Nagler is Physiatrist-in-Chief, Department of Physical Medicine and Rehabilitation, New York Hospital-Cornell Medical Center.

DR. NORMAN ORENTREICH   ° Hair °   Chapter 11

Dr. Norman Orentreich is Director of the Orentreich Medical Group and Associate Clinical Professor of Dermatology, New York University School of Medicine.

DR. JAMES C. PARKES II   ° Hands °   Chapter 10

Dr. Parkes is Attending Orthopedic Surgeon at Roosevelt Hospital, New York. He teaches at Columbia Presbyterian Hospital. Dr. Parkes is also Orthopedic Surgeon for the New York Mets baseball team.

BARBARA PEARLMAN   ° Exercise °   Chapters 2, 40

Barbara Pearlman is a former dancer, who now teaches exercise in New York. She has an exercise studio, and also calls on private homes and offices. She is the author of *Barbara Pearlman's Dance Exercises* (Doubleday/Dolphin).

DR. SAMUEL M. PECK   ° Skin °   Chapter 7

Dr. Peck is Professor of Dermatology Emeritus, Mount Sinai School of Medicine, New York. He is also Director Emeritus of Mount Sinai School of Medicine, and currently a consultant there.

DR. A. BENEDICT RIZZUTI   ° Eyes °   Chapter 8

Dr. Rizzuti is Consultant Ophthalmologist, New York Eye and Ear Infirmary, and Methodist Hospital, Brooklyn; and Clinical Professor of Ophthalmology, New York Medical College. Dr. Rizzuti is also a board member of the International Eye Foundation.

DR. ELIZABETH ROBERTS   ° Feet °   Chapter 35

Dr. Roberts is a podiatrist practicing in New York City. She is also Professor Emeritus, New York College of Podiatric Medicine, and author of *On Your Feet* (Rodale Press).

DR. JEAN W. SALEH   ° Stomach °   Chapter   2

Dr. Saleh is Assistant Attending Physician and Associate in Medicine, College of Physicians and Surgeons, Columbia University, and gastroenterologist at St. Luke's Hospital, New York.

DR. RICHARD O. SCHUSTER ° Running °   Chapter 36

Dr. Schuster is Professor of Biomechanics, New York College of Podiatric Medicine. He is also a specialist in the field of orthotics, the science of running, and consultant on the design of running and sports shoes.

DR. FRANCES MERITT STERN ° Weight Control °
Chapter 32

Dr. Stern is Associate Professor of Psychology at Kean College and Director of the Institute for Behavioral Awareness in Springfield, New Jersey. She is coauthor, with Ruth S. Hoch, of *Mind Trips To Help You Lose Weight* (Playboy Press).

DR. DIANE G. TANENBAUM   ° Skin °   Chapter 40

Dr. Tanenbaum is Associate Professor of Dermatology, New York University, and Attending Physician, Lenox Hill Hospital in New York.

DORIS TOBIAS   ° Weight Control °   Chapter 33

Doris Tobias writes a wine and restaurant column for *Women's Wear Daily,* and wine and food features for *W.* She is also coauthor, with Mary Merris, of *The Golden Lemon* (Athenaeum).

ELOISE R. TRESCHER, R.D. ° Nutrition ° Chapters 13–29

Mrs. Trescher was founder of the Nutrition Clinic, the Johns Hopkins Hospital, Baltimore, Maryland, and former member of the faculty of the Johns Hopkins University Medical School. She is also coauthor of the first Manual of Applied Nutrition for Johns Hopkins Hospital, consultant nutritionist for *House & Garden,* and in private practice.

DR. MARY CATHERINE TYSON ° General Health ° Chapter 12

Dr. Tyson is an internist and Assistant Physican, Hematology, at Mount Sinai Hospital. She helped to start the blood bank there in 1940. Together with her late husband, Dr. Tyson, she wrote *The Psychology of Successful Weight Control* (Nelson Hall).

DR. NEWTON K. WESLEY ° Contact Lenses ° Chapter 8

Dr. Wesley is an optometrist who pioneered the development of the multi-focal contact lens. He is chairman of the National Eye Research Foundation, a non-profit organization engaged in vision research.

DR. LENORE R. ZOHMAN ° Heart ° Chapter 1

Dr. Zohman is Director of Cardiopulmonary Rehabilitation, Montefiore Hospital, New York, and Associate Professor of Cardiology, Albert Einstein College of Medicine. She is also a member of the Exercise Committee of the American Heart Association.

ACKNOWLEDGMENTS

The editors of *House & Garden* would like to thank all the doctors and experts who gave up so much of their valuable time to our interviewers. Some of the busiest people in the world, they shared their knowledge and insights, answering questions and confirming facts for us with great generosity, both in and out of office hours. We were privileged to have access to such distinguished and experienced professionals.

We would also like to thank the members of our staff who met and talked to the experts: Beverly Russell, Senior Editor, Jane Ellis, Wine and Food Editor, and Paula Rice Jackson, Beauty and Health Editor; also our outside contributors, Elin Schoen, Naomi Barry, Pamela Markham, and Doris Tobias.

INTRODUCTION

Today, more and more people are realizing that being healthy involves every aspect of living—from the food we eat, the exercise we take, and the air we breathe, to the way we use our minds.

All these elements of life concern *House & Garden* readers, and this book is a selection of our most popular features on these subjects. *Total Health* contains the advice and opinions of top doctors and experts in the field of health and fitness about how to handle our bodies and our minds. Their guidelines will help you make the right decisions today about taking care of yourself and your family.

The book offers what amounts to free consultations with many of the best-known doctors in America. Experienced nutritionists present food basics and offer suggestions that will help you and your family eat right, with recipes for you to follow; and we have also collected the diet and fitness secrets from five world-famous spas for you to use at home. Finally, we focus on techniques for a healthy mind, without which you cannot expect your body to function at its best.

The information in this book will, we hope, be a permanent guide for you to consult as you need it, helping you to help yourself lead a happier, healthier life.

The editors of *House & Garden*
December 1977

Part One

A HEALTHY BODY FROM HEAD TO TOE

In this section, world-famous specialists check out parts of your body, explaining their growth, functions, and how to keep them healthy. Their consultations can help you look after yourself better and understand a little more about how your body works.

Chapter 1

AFFAIRS OF THE HEART

The heart is our most vital piece of organic equipment. In recent years, medical research has revealed many of its most intricate secrets. At the same time, statistics reveal that cardiovascular disease is the major cause of death in the United States of America. Two of the best-known cardiologists in America have been consulted here to give their advice and personal tips for keeping your heart healthy—and that's the gift of a good long life.

HEARTS AND CHARTS

The heart is a pump. It has the responsibility of pumping blood around the body, providing the various organs with nourishment. Most of the time we don't think about it; it beats away, according to our activities, and we probably pay more attention to it as a symbol of love, joy, and generosity ("sweetheart," "light-hearted," "big-hearted") than as our most vital piece of organic equipment.

Except when something happens to it. There are some unchangeable risk factors that affect a healthy heart—heredity, getting older, and being male (women before menopause have far fewer heart attacks than men). Other risk factors *can* be controlled: high blood pressure can be treated; you can stop smoking; you can keep your weight down; you can try to minimize stress; and you can exercise.

It's a familiar list and difficult for most of us to adhere to, except for one requirement—exercise. This is because a wonderfully simple technique of exercise—that anyone can do, anywhere, anytime—has been developed specifically for heart health by Dr. Lenore R. Zohman, with other exercise cardiologists, and endorsed by the American Heart Association.

Dr. Zohman is Director of Cardiopulmonary Rehabilitation at Montefiore Hospital, New York, and Associate Professor of Cardiology at the Albert Einstein College of Medicine. She is a Fellow of the American College of Cardiology, and a member of the Exercise Committee of the American Heart Association.

"Until recently," Dr. Zohman explains, "it was difficult to test people's ability to be active. It was not possible to do a dynamic examination or an electrocardiogram on a moving patient—people were examined lying down. With the latest developments in equipment, we can now measure people while they are moving. This science of exercise programing has been worked out as a consequence. We test people's heart rate, blood pressure, and oxygen while they use a treadmill or a bicycle. Depending on the results, we can prescribe how much exercise a person should do to maintain a healthy heart.

"Here's how it works: There is an amount of exercise sufficient to condition the muscles and cardiovascular system, leading to physical fitness, but it is not overly strenuous. That is, there is a target zone in which your heart rate increases enough to achieve fitness, but not too much to exceed safe limits. The name of the game is finding your target zone—your target heart rate zone.

"Each individual's target zone is between 70 and 85 percent of his own maximum attainable heart rate. Above 85 percent, the circulation finds it increasingly difficult to supply oxygen rapidly to the exercising muscles—hence you puff and pant to try to take in more oxygen." Each person has a different target zone. You can either find this out by

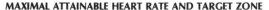

MAXIMAL ATTAINABLE HEART RATE AND TARGET ZONE

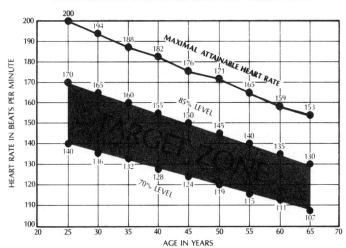

AGE IN YEARS

This figure shows that as we grow older, the highest heart rate which can be reached during all-out effort falls. These numerical values are "average" values for age. Note that one-third of the population may differ from these values. It is quite possible that a normal 50-year-old man may have a maximum heart rate of 195 or that a 30-year-old man might have a maximum of only 168. The same limitations apply to the 70 per cent and 85 per cent of maximum lines.

taking an exercise stress-test under supervision of a specially trained doctor, or you can estimate it roughly by using the maximal attainable heart rate and target zone chart. Example: A twenty-year-old-man has a maximal heart rate of 200. His target zone would then be 140 (70 percent) to 170 (85 percent) beats per minute heart rate. A sixty-five-year-old man with a maximal attainable heart rate of 150 beats per minute, would have a target zone of 107 (70 percent) to 130 (85 percent) beats per minute.

Once you have found your target zone, all you have to do is find exercise that gets your heart rate up to that zone for approximately 20–30 minutes, 3 times a week. To determine whether you are in your target zone, take your pulse (it's easiest either at the wrist or at the side of the neck). Plan the program so that there is a warm-up and cool-down period of about 5–10 minutes to adjust circulation. Make sure that your exercise is aerobic, that is, you take in oxygen in the same amount that you use it up, so there is a balance. For example, jog instead of run—puffing and panting like a sprinter is *not* helping your heart, and merely exhausts you.

Ideally, before anyone starts an exercise program, Dr. Zohman recommends a consultation with a doctor. And if possible, take the exercise stress-test to find your target zone. If this is not possible in your area, and if you are healthy, it is probably reasonable to assume that your maximum attainable heart rate is 220 minus your age, and and that your target zone is 70–85 percent of that maximum. Whether you exercise or not, you should definitely have your blood pressure taken once a year. There is a big campaign all over the country to encourage people to do this—because you can have hypertension (high blood pressure) and not feel a thing. Your doctor can see it though—and the earlier you catch it, the better for your heart.

ONE MAN'S HEART—Dr. Denton Cooley

"I'm fifty-seven right now and I fully expect to live to be ninety. I think that all of my ancestors would have lived that long had they taken better care of themselves." Denton Cooley, M.D., is Surgeon-in-Chief of the Texas Heart Institute and Surgical Consultant to St. Luke's Episcopal and Texas Children's Hospitals, Houston. His numerous awards include the René Lériche Award of the International Society of Surgery 1967 for the most outstanding contribution to heart surgery during the previous two years. Five years ago, Denton Cooley, who has done many thousands of open heart operations, had the courage to undertake surgery implanting the first artificial heart into a dying patient. He strives to prolong life—his own, his family's, his friends', his patients'. His patients, whom he treats as friends, come to him from all parts of the world.

Dr. Cooley looks at the most forty-five—suntanned, slim and incredibly handsome. If you didn't know who he was, you might think he was a professional athlete. In fact, he plays tennis, golf, basketball, is a horseback rider, and a double bass player in The Heartbeats, an orchestra made up mostly of physicians at the Texas Heart Institute, of which he was a founder. "I just sort of picked it up, I've not been playing long. It's fun, but I'm not sure it's good for my hands, these old double basses are brutal on your fingers and give you blisters."

Recreation is essential to his live-longer philosophy. "I'm blessed with a good ancestry and a good track record of health in both my mother's parents and my father's parents and that, to me, is a very good insurance policy. But I've always believed in a balanced life. Work, rest, and recreation. Work is vital to a long and healthy life and in adding meaning to your life. Rest, too. But it doesn't matter how you budget your sleep time, that's up to the individual. You don't need to sleep eight hours continuously, but you must have adequate rest. Recreation is just as necessary. You've got to have some diversion from day to day—work, rest, and recreation programs to keep yourself in good shape. I believe one must think about all three and allot time for each."

No day for Dr. Cooley passes without some exercise, in addition to the walking marathons through hospital corridors, seeing patients. He's often at the Heart Institute eighteen hours a day, on his feet from 6 A.M. performing up to fifteen operations, checking on postoperative cases, seeing future ones, talking to relatives. And always outpacing junior colleagues with his energy. "The question of exercise isn't just to keep the weight down. It keeps all the muscles including the heart muscle in tone and this is a very important safeguard. By exercising, stressing the heart to the proper degree, we develop collateral coronary circulation, so that if one of the major vessels of the heart does get in trouble, the collateral vessels will take over the support of that injured part.

"A lot of things are derived from exercise that helps to keep the legs and hips in good tone. Low-back problems are the bane of middle-aged people, particularly. They usually come from relaxation of the abdominal and pelvic muscles, often through sedentary occupation. So if you keep the major muscle mass from the waist down in shape, you've gone a long way toward cardiovascular health and to keeping general health as well. You don't have to go into a vigorous time-consuming program like some men have of jogging 30 minutes a day. Frankly, I just can't spare the time for that, so I run in place in the bedroom or dressing room, or hop on one foot 50 times and then do the same on the other. If you do that twice a day in the space of less than 5 minutes each session, then you've got as good exercise almost as playing an hour of singles tennis."

Curiously, however hard we try, sometimes extra pounds appear and Dr. Cooley says he's no exception. This is where diet comes in. "I'm one of those people who really take an assessment of their physique before the mirror while shaving in the morning, and if it looks like there's getting to be a little middle-aged spread, then I'll skip a meal or two, or just not eat so much. And I keep a bathroom scales and keep my weight where I want it, 185, and I'm 6 feet 4, which seems okay for my physique."

Being the proper weight for your size is intimately connected with a healthy heart. If you are heavy, that doesn't necessarily mean you're unhealthy or going to die prematurely, but the more weight you carry around, the more the demand on the circulation. "The same heart size, the same blood vessel setup," explains Dr. Cooley, "may have to supply twice as much tissue. Of course the heart will adjust to this and it will enlarge, but it's clear that overweight people come to suffer from complications of all sorts from circulation and cardiac disease. I'm not a stickler for a strict diet and I think there are too many faddists in medicine who put patients on strict low cholesterol programs. I'm more inclined to recommend appropriate caloric intake depending on weight and size. But some rather extensive studies show that high levels of saturated fats—those that are solid at room temperature and usually come from animal sources—contribute to high levels of cholesterol in the blood stream and this is inclined to produce changes in blood vessels, which lead to coronary disease.

"We can't eliminate fats entirely from the diet; they're our principal source of energy, providing more than twice as much caloric value gram per gram as carbohydrates and proteins, but the types of fats are very important. We should go for fish and fowl and vegetable oils—the polyunsaturated fats that are liquid at room temperature—rather than animal fats. Of course milk is good nourishment for children, but many individuals persist in a high milk intake throughout adulthood, particularly whole milk with cream and high butterfat content. I drink skim milk, though I get most of the milk intake I need with my standard lunch of soup and ice cream. Eggs? Well, we found a substitute for butter in margarine and it's possible that we'll find a substitute for eggs if we need to break the habit, but I'm not sure that they're so harmful. There's cholesterol in them of course, but they're low calorie and if one takes exercise and restricts intake of starches and carbohydrates, the amount of cholesterol in an egg is not going to affect the serum cholesterol. I eat, I guess, a dozen eggs a week myself, at breakfast and other meals, and I've had no real serious concern about that."

What about heart checkups? "I think they are extremely important. One useful test is the exercise-of-stress electrocardiogram using the mechanical treadmill device. You or I could go and have a cardiogram made while lying on a couch and it would probably be pretty normal. But if you walked at a fast rate, ten miles an hour on a slight incline, then changes in the electrocardiogram may appear, reflecting the fact that there is a cardiac problem in the heart under stressful conditions."

If you can work out ways to beat daily strains from

building up, so much the better. Dr. Cooley has stereo music
playing during surgery. Often he'll take a pineapple yoghurt
break between complicated operations. But he never resorts
to smoking. "Smoking and alcohol in large quantities have an
adverse effect on cardiac rhythm. There's no question that
emotions, anxiety, and stress have an effect, too. Our involuntary nervous system produces hormones through the adrenal
glands during periods of stress, which may push the blood
pressure up. There are various things that fall under the
heading of mental hygiene to cope with this. Meditation
might be worthwhile and helpful, but it's not my cup of tea.
I believe more in playing a little tennis and being with the
family, getting out of town for a day and going to my ranch.
I get a great deal of relaxation through my family, five
daughters, and their friends."

Dr. Cooley raised $10 million privately through patients
and philanthropists to build the twenty-nine-story Texas
Heart Institute and is constantly campaigning for more funds
for trainees, better health care and research. He confidently
predicts: "In the next twenty years we'll see a practical
artificial heart with an external power source; the internal
power source may be an impossible dream but we'll learn
something from all the experiments. We're doing things that
were undreamed of in surgery ten years ago. Patients who
were completely incapacitated or at death's door are now
completely rehabilitated. It's an entirely new world."

What was learned from the heart transplant "era"? One of
the interesting by-products was the changing attitude toward
the heart and life in general. "From the beginning of human
knowledge too much has been ascribed to the heart—our
emotions, our fears, our sadness, happiness. I think it's
because it's the only organ that you can actually see or feel
working. But we shouldn't think of it as a touch-me-not. It is
just another organ in our body and should be treated as such.
The best concept of the body is that it resembles a household. The brain is the master of the house. If there is an
anatomical seat for the soul it must be in the brain; that is

where those intangible things such as one's mind, spirit, and personality must reside, not in the heart. What is the heart anyway? It's a very simple thing, it just pumps blood, therefore its function is simple compared to the liver or the kidney. The heart being the center of all activity is a mistaken idea. If people knew more about their bodies and their body functions, they'd be better equipped to cope with the situations that arise every day. The experience with heart transplants proved to everyone that the heart of one person could serve another master—evidence for that is to be seen in the patients who have lived five years after having had a heart transplant."

Back in his comfortable office in the Texas Heart Institute Dr. Cooley has this quotation from André Gide alongside a color portrait of his heart transplant team: "Man cannot discover new oceans unless he has the courage to lose sight of the shore." Dr. Cooley plunged all the way into uncharted depths of surgery. He has emerged as a heroic lifesaver. He repeats: "We've got to strive to prolong life. No one is immortal. You know you're going to die but you just don't want to do it today, tomorrow, or even next month."

HEART PICK-ME-UPS

Some people do not like, or do not have the time, to exercise. Dr. Zohman has some ideas for you—solutions that are easy to accomplish since they concern your day-to-day living, and that are sufficient to get your heart up into that target zone and thus achieve the exercise your heart needs.

Go dancing

Fitness dancing to music is excellent for the heart—and it's fun. Go-go dancing, rock, modern dance, even a continuous program of ballroom dancing, all raise your heart rate and do your heart (and social life) good.

Do housework

To reach target levels, bunch together several active tasks such as a big vacuuming job, scrubbing a floor, washing blinds, for no longer than a 20–30 minute period. Warm up first by washing dishes or dusting and cool down by putting dishes away or folding clothes. In this way your house is clean, you've saved money—and helped your heart! *(Don't* do all the housework in one day, so you end up totally exhausted. Remember this new technique of exercise is a 3-times-a-week program, without exhausting you or straining your muscles.)

Climb stairs

Walk briskly up and down two or three flights—not so fast that you pant. This is excellent heart exercise. A study was recently done of an office building where everyone who worked above the 17th floor had to walk up the stairs. Those working below 17 could take elevators. When they tested the physical condition of the employees, those who worked above the 17th floor were much fitter than those who worked below!

Work in the garden

Collect together the more strenuous activities such as digging, weeding, or mowing, and do them consecutively so that you maintain your target zone for 20–30 minutes. Find warm-up and cool-down activities such as picking flowers or repotting plants.

All these activities are part of daily life. If you prefer, a program of brisk walking, jogging, swimming, bicycling, or skipping rope will achieve the same results—good heart exercise with the right oxygen balance, no panting or exhaustion—your own personal fitness program.

This simple "science of exercise," worked out by Dr. Zohman and her colleagues with the endorsement of the American Heart Association, will make you feel better, look better, improve your heart rate, and create that feeling of well-being that springs from a healthy and happy heart.

Chapter 2

THE INSIDE STORY

The stomach is hardly the most glamorous part of the human body. Most people only think about it when it gets larger than is acceptable in a weight-conscious world, or when it starts acting up—there is no way of ignoring that most common of stomach complaints, indigestion, for instance. But the stomach is really a fascinating organ, and works in all sorts of ingenious ways to keep you healthy and energetic.

Did you imagine the stomach as a large cavern somewhere behind your belly-button, rather like a washing machine, in which food gets whirled about and ejected? Wrong. It's at rib level, with its upper end just below the heart. Did you know that you have about 3,000 taste buds in your mouth, and that before you can taste anything, the substance must be moistened by your salivary glands? Did you know that the way your stomach rumbles can tell people things? Doctors are now learning to diagnose stomach problems by listening to the various noises emerging from it. Did you ever guess that your liver, the largest and most versatile gland in the body, has about 500 chemical roles to play in detoxifying food and turning it into fuel? Americans spend over $218 million a year for laxatives and $127 million for antacids—but did you know both problems are often preventable without recourse to pills or powders? And had you any idea that about 80 percent of indigestion has no organic bearing whatsoever, i.e., is simply to do with the way you eat rather than with the state of your stomach?

Well, unless you're a professional gastroenterologist you're never going to know precisely what goes on in those mysterious intestinal passages. You probably would prefer not to know anyway. What you really *do* want to know is how to avoid stomach troubles—and that means asking certain key questions of someone who has spent his life understanding and curing them—Dr. Jean Saleh, Assistant Attending Physician, College of Physicians and Surgeons, Columbia University, New York, and gastroenterologist at St. Luke's Hospital. His answers may help clear up some of the confusion and make you more sympathetic to that under-praised part of your anatomy.

Q. What is acid indigestion?
A. "There is no such thing. 'Acid indigestion' does not mean anything. Your stomach secretes acid in order to break down food. That is normal. If you have pernicious anemia, you will have less acid than normal, if any at all. If you have a duodenal ulcer, you will have more acid than normal. The stomach has a built-in defense mechanism, mucus, to buffer the acidity it produces. If you have too much acid for the buffer to work, then you may damage the lining of the stomach, producing gastritis, inflammation of the stomach, or ulcers. This has nothing to do with indigestion—it has only to do with excess acid. Antacids may temporarily help with these conditions, but a doctor should be consulted.

"Eighty percent of indigestion has no organic bearing whatsoever. Indigestion may mean anything from delayed emptying of the stomach excess gas, abdominal discomfort, to nausea. The stomach normally empties from an hour to two hours, depending on the quality of the foods. Fat takes much more time to get out of the stomach than protein or sugar; sometimes as much as an hour longer. Remember that the stomach is not just a reservoir or pouch; it works on the food, mixing it with acid, contracting up and down in order to make it smooth and digestible. Indigestion occurs when this function is inhibited or exaggerated—for instance, if you eat too fast, fail to chew, are unable to relax. The stomach protests by producing spasms, and you may feel bloated because it cannot empty effectively."

Q. When people diet successfully, they often say they feel less hungry. Is that because the stomach shrinks?
A. "It's hard to say the stomach shrinks when you go on a diet, because nobody has ever documented that. People who are very obese, consuming 15,000 to 25,000 calories a day, have enlarged stomachs, since the elastic part of the wall distends to some extent. On a diet, the stomach will return to its normal size. If you go on a semi-starvation diet, then perhaps you may have some shrinking, because you are losing so much protein. But this is only in very drastic situations, and not well proven.

"When people say they no longer feel hungry, that usually has nothing to do with the size of the stomach. If you have not eaten for some length of time, you may experience what we call a hunger pang, when the stomach starts contracting. But hunger is usually a psychological effect just as is feeling 'full.' A normal individual will eat a steak and probably feel full very quickly. The impression of fullness, however, doesn't mean only that the pouch of your stomach is filled with food all the way up, but also that you are satisfied with the number of calories you have consumed; because you have some set point in your hypothalamus where all the centers of hunger and satiety reside, registering satisfaction.

"For an overweight person, this register in the hypothalamus is somehow not working. If you ask obese people how they feel when hungry, they find it difficult to answer. They don't point to their stomachs, where normal people feel hunger pains—they point to the upper part of their chest or their throat, anywhere. Their hunger is not identifiable, and that means it is largely psychological. And that is why they will not experience what normal people know as 'fullness.' "

Q. Why does the stomach sometimes rumble?
A. "Before eating, rumbles may be due to excessive spasm—that is, the stomach moving air and secretions. Because even if we don't eat, we are secreting fluid from the blood into the intestines. We swallow air, and air comes from the combustion of food and cells themselves. There is always action in the stomach—for instance, if we don't eat for a week, we still have some bowel movements. When the stomach is coping with too much air or liquid, you will hear it on the outside as a rumble. As soon as you ingest food, this situation will calm down.

"Swallowing too much air can cause burps. This may occur if you are nervous, working under stress, or have some emotional problem. In these situations, you may experience an increase in the spastic ability of the gastro-intestinal tract. But burping is also a defense mechanism and is perfectly acceptable."

Q. Are vitamin supplements good for the stomach?
A. "There are no vitamin supplements specifically good for the stomach. A well-balanced diet in terms of protein, fat, carbohydrate, minerals, and vitamins is what your body needs. If you eat properly, you don't need vitamin supplements. If you take only vitamins, without eating, they won't help at all, because vitamins are what we call coenzymes in terms of metabolism of food. They will act if you bring something to them. Eating only vitamins is like going to a gas station and pouring the gas on the floor. They need a vehicle, and the vehicle is food. Iron alone, for instance, goes right through your body—iron *plus* protein builds red cells. (That does not mean you have to take iron at the same time as a meal, however. Iron is transformed better, and absorbed better, taken separately.)"

EXPERT TIPS FOR A HEALTHY STOMACH

Dr. Saleh suggests the following guidelines to keep your stomach in good working order:

1. Eat in a relaxed environment. Try to avoid business luncheons and dinners, which give the stomach twice as much work, through stress as well as poor eating.

2. Chew carefully. (It used to be said that you should chew each mouthful 25 times!)

3. Avoid an excess of alcohol, smoking, coffee, and spices. All can alter the lining of the stomach and its function. (Antacids only relieve excess acidity for about 45 minutes.)

4. Put fiber in your diet. It has been shown in recent years that fiber may decrease the possibility of constipation, and prevent more severe disorders.

5. If you have pain consistently after eating, see a doctor.

EASY STOMACH EXERCISES

"You can help your stomach every minute of the day," says exercise expert Barbara Pearlman. "Just pull it in towards your back whenever you can remember—walking, sitting down, resting. Don't make an effort to let go; it will go back of its own accord. And don't hold in your breath. Just move with it tucked in whenever you can. This also automatically strengthens your back." She also suggests these floor exercises to firm up the muscles.

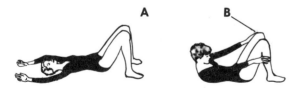

Lie on back, knees bent, soles of feet parallel and about 10 inches apart; arms extended on floor over head, palms facing upward (a). Inhale deeply as you lift upper body off floor. Arms simultaneously swing forward (b). Hold for 2 slow counts, then exhale as you release to original position. Repeat 8 times.

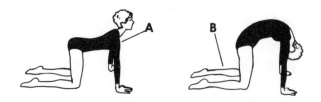

Begin on hands and knees, back sunk in, head up (a). Inhale deeply. Drop head, round back, as you tightly contract your abdominal muscles (b). Hold for 3 slow counts, then exhale and slowly resume original position. Repeat 8 times.

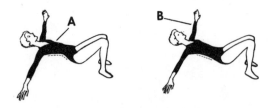

Lie on back, knees bent, feet flat on floor, arms at shoulder level (a). Contract your abdominal muscles as you press your back firmly against the floor (b). Hold the contraction for 5 slow counts, then release. Repeat 10 times.

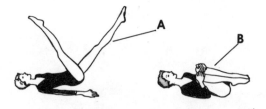

Lie on floor with legs extending upward, toes pointed, arms resting at sides (a). Keeping abdominal muscles contracted, and back flat against floor, scissor kick legs forward and back 8 times. Then bend knees and draw them close to your chest (b). Hold 4 counts. Repeat sequence 3 times.

Chapter 3

PUTTING YOUR BACK INTO IT

It's your backbone that holds you up—and has undergone a great deal of strain in the process, as we evolved from four-legged creatures to vertical-spined humans. Maybe it's not so surprising that 1 in every 3 Americans has experienced severe backache more than once during his or her lifetime. No wonder, either, according to the U.S. Bureau of Statistics, backache is the second most frequent cause of absenteeism from work (the first being the common cold and influenza). The question is, what can help it? You can't see backache; you can't hear it. But you sure would like to know what to do about it. Relax, and read on. You'll be in the hands of an expert.

"OH, MY POOR BACK!"

It usually happens one of two ways. One's dramatic. The other's subtle. Bending over to pick up a pencil that dropped on the floor and not being able to straighten up again for the searing pain in your back. Or waking up on a bright morning to find an intractable current of discomfort coming from the low back. The statistics describing the occurrence of low-back pain for Americans are staggering: 70,000,000 have experienced a severe backache more than once in their life; 7,000,000 receive medical treatment of some kind for low-back pain every day of the year; 2,000,000 more Americans are added to either of these two categories each year. Which means that 1 out of 3 Americans suffers from low-back pain and back-related problems. In most people's book, that's an epidemic.

DR. FINNESON ON LOW-BACK PAIN

Bernard E. Finneson, M.D., is Chief of Neurosurgery and Director of the Low Back Pain Clinic of the Crozer-Chester Medical Center in Chester, Pennsylvania, as well as Chief of Neurosurgery at two other hospitals. He is Associate Professor of Neurological Surgery at Hahnemann Medical College in Philadelphia where he received his M.D. in 1948. A Philadelphia internship was followed by residencies in neuropsychiatry and neurosurgery. His personal and professional concerns have been the treatment and study of the myriad causes of low-back pain that afflicts so many.

Dr. Finneson describes low-back pain as a result, in part, of the evolutionary process. Your posture is erect. You walk on two feet instead of four. Varicose veins, flat feet, hemorrhoids, and abdominal hernias have also been described as being part of the price for walking upright. Only man stands erect and the resultant forward curvature of his lower spine, which differentiates him from all other primates, is also the cause of his backaches.

At birth the human spine resembles an elongated curve like a "C," but stretched. At maturity it is no longer straight, but more like an "S" dipped forward in the abdominal or lower back area, curving backward in the chest section, and then forward again as it stretches upward into the neck where it supports the weight of the head. The center of gravity is shifted forward, where it is balanced by the muscles of the buttocks, a uniquely human attribute. The spine is like a system of building blocks piled atop each other with shock absorbers placed in between each block. Another system of muscles, ligaments, and tendons acts as a set of guy wires which prevent the column from toppling.

The area below the rib cage, the five massive vertebrae of the lumbar region, is both the powerhouse of the spine and its most vulnerable, sensitive part. The lumbar region acts as a fulcrum for the rest of the body—the legs and torso. The spinal cord, which is safely encased inside the spinal column for 95 percent of its length, ends in a compact but loose array of threadlike nerves at the base of the spine. That's another considerable reason for low-back pain: irritated, unprotected nerve endings. A third is the natural aging of the intervertebrals, or spinal disks, which act as cushions between the bony parts of the spine. Considering the number of stresses and pressures affecting the spine, it's a miracle that it isn't more sensitive than it is.

To many people, back pain is associated with a "slipped disk." The spinal disks give the spine the mobility to bend forward, stretch backward, twist from side to side. They are the largest in the lumbar region where they're exposed to the greatest pressure due to stress. The disks have a gel-like consistency, which spreads stress and pressure on the vertebrae uniformly. They act as transmitters of forces on the bony part of the spine just like shock absorbers. A disk can rupture and send fibrous tissue into the spinal column and its surrounding area, causing dreadful pain. But it is very important to remember that there are other possible reasons for a severe pain—so don't assume it's a disk.

Low back pain is often the result of overexertion and nothing more. Most of us can tell the difference between this kind of backache and something more serious. Vigorous physical exercise such as tennis, golf, or horseback riding, which stresses the structure of the low back, may result in stiffness, soreness, a dull ache. It goes away in a day or two and it usually happens when it's the first physical activity we've had for a while. But if after three days the pain persists, it's time to call a doctor.

THE FINNESON PREVENTIVE PLAN

Literally thousands of patients suffering from low-back dysfunctions come to Dr. Finneson's clinic for help. After tests and examinations, he starts them on a regimen of daily exercise designed to strengthen the abdomen and the muscles of the low back. "Daily exercise is a must. The effort is useless without this daily physical demand," says Dr. Finneson.

For those of us who suffer occasional or mild low-back pain, Dr. Finneson offers preventive advice. "After the age of thirty-five, there's a change in the quality of muscle tone that's similar to the difference between a rubber band and a piece of string. Youth compensates for its own excesses of physical activity. With age, a respect, an awareness, and a program of care to maintain muscle tone become increasingly important." It's easy to follow his advice. Take 5 minutes before you go out on the tennis court that fine June morning and spend it doing exercises that prepare you and limber you up. See his effective detensing, preparatory exercises on the next page.

After the game, take a hot shower or preferably a bath and soak. And, if you're really fortunate, have a massage. It can be especially helpful the first few times you work out. After the muscles are accustomed to the movement you can eliminate it. But the half-hour soak is always a good idea. Should you find that there is stiffness the next day, take a hot bath before and after work and one more before going to bed. However, if the stiffness in the low back is so great that walking and moving are downright disagreeable, go to bed. Bed rest is essential, as it literally takes the load off your back. If lying on your back is uncomfortable, a ¾-inch-thick piece of plywood under the mattress can help make it firmer. Or roll pillows and place them under your knees to help press the small of your back flat. You may find that lying on your side with knees slightly bent is the most comfortable. Don't lie on your stomach, however. That natural curve at the base of the spine will curve inward even more and increase the pain. Once you're up and about wear low-heeled shoes for a while.

Some people find that cold treatments work better for them than heat. Dr. Finneson's recipe for ice-lollipops: Fill an empty orange-juice tin with water and when it's partially frozen insert a Popsicle stick or tongue depressor. The lollipop slips out of the can when warm water is run over it. The ice is applied directly to the skin until it has been numbed, then applied 5 seconds more. The effect is a topical anesthetic which relieves pain and lasts. Dr. Finneson suggests that as a rule, for low-back pain, try heat first, then cold. One should work. An aspirin or two can also relieve the pain, as will the new aspirin substitutes like Tylenol or Datril.

One more word about exercising. *Do not* exercise during a period of acute low-back pain. "Working it out" is a myth and can result in further muscle spasm. Always check with your doctor, physiotherapist, or orthopedist before embarking on an exercise if you know that your bad back involves more than passing stiffness. And watch your weight. That lithe, supple spine is affected by the amount it carries, so keep an eye on the scale.

Do the warm-up before every physically exerting activity:

1. a. Lie flat on back on floor with legs extended.
   b. Raise arms slowly above head while inhaling slowly.
   c. Allow arms to return to sides while exhaling slowly.
   d. Relax entire body.
   e. Repeat 10 times.

2. a. Inhale slowly while tightening all body muscles (clench fists tightly to sides, squeeze legs together, tighten buttocks, etc.).
   b. Exhale and relax all muscles; close eyes.
   c. Repeat 10 times.

Chapter 4

FEELING IT IN YOUR BONES

Normally we don't spend much time thinking about our bones. Sometimes they ache; sometimes they are stiff; some-times you wish they were different (it being the fashion to desire "good bones" in a face); sometimes they tell you things (think of the chill that runs through your bones when you are scared of something); but most of the time we tend to concentrate on the more external parts of the body, because they are what *show*.

But your bones hold you up, move you around, keep body and soul together. Made of mineral and protein, they are the supporting part of the body, and like the muscles, heart, and almost all parts of the body, they work best when they are used regularly.

WHAT CAN HAPPEN TO YOUR BONES?

The most common problem with bones is osteoporosis, or softening of the bones. "This means the bones become brittle and break easily," says Dr. William G. Hamilton. Dr. Hamilton is Orthopedist for the New York City Ballet, Orthopedic Surgeon at Roosevelt Hospital, New York, and Instructor in Orthopedics, Columbia University College of Physicians and Surgeons. He is a Fellow of the American College of Surgeons, member of the American Academy of Orthopedic Surgeons, and has published various papers in the field of children's orthopedics. "Constantly during your lifetime," he explains, "there is a turnover of calcium, phosphorus, and other minerals in your bones. The minerals are taken out of the bone and then replaced. But as you get older, for some reason the mineral goes out and is not replaced. There are two possible causes of this. One is disuse—inactivity leads to premature softening of the bones. For instance, when you put a limb in a cast for a fracture, this causes a softening of the bones. Of course in this situation it is only temporary, but disuse has that effect on the bones. The other possible cause, we now think, is poor diet—not enough calcium and vitamin D."

Dr. Hamilton says there are two vital questions you should ask yourself if you want to keep your bones good and strong.

Are you a weekend athlete?

Don't be. Dr. Hamilton says that the single most important thing for a healthy body—bones, muscles, and joints—is regular physical activity. "It always comes back to that," he emphasizes. "The biggest problem in modern society is disuse. The skeletal system responds to activity, and the pull of the muscles helps bones stay strong. This was proved with the astronauts. It was found that they suffered a severe loss of calcium from their bones when they were in a weightless condition. In order to prevent this, special exercises had to be devised to keep the mineral in their bones."

Keep active, Dr. Hamilton urges. "People are inactive for thirteen days and then on the fourteenth day they go out and try to make up for all that inactivity. That's the wrong approach. I see patients all the time with strains and pulls and back pains simply because they tried to make up for their inactivity all at once. Don't be a weekend athlete. What's important is regular activity on a daily basis. Even walking to work is better than sitting all day. Try bicycle riding—that's excellent exercise—far better than playing tennis once a month. Activity keeps bones strong."

Are you drinking enough milk?

According to Dr. Hamilton, it is now thought that diet plays a much more important part in bone health than was previously believed. "In fact, we're beginning to feel that softening of the bones in old people is not osteoporosis alone but also osteomalacia—rickets in adults—caused by the inadequate intake of calcium and vitamin D. Most doctors now feel that you should have the equivalent of almost a quart of skimmed milk a day in calcium intake throughout your life. You don't need the fat of whole milk, but skimmed milk contains the calcium, vitamin D, and protein that your bones need. People think milk is just for children—that is not true.

"We recommend drinking a quart of skimmed milk a day or its equivalent in yoghurt or cottage cheese for people with softening of the bones. And for everyone else, as close to a quart as you can. Milk is simply the most convenient way of taking in calcium—calcium tablets are often poorly absorbed. By drinking enough skimmed milk from childhood on, you will keep your calcium intake up all your life and keep your bones strong."

Before your bones start creaking at the thought, here's something to cheer you up. Dr. Hamilton is orthopedist for the New York City Ballet, and if you've ever longed for your bones to move as effortlessly as a ballet dancer's, listen to what he says about these particular clients: "A dancer's body is at its finest. Their injuries are usually not serious—pulls and strains and injured knees—but serious for them of course because their career is threatened. They are in such perfect condition, and yet they push themselves so hard that they all have problems. It's part of dancing—to hurt. In fact, most of the star dancers will say that they hurt off and on during their whole career."

So when you next watch Natalia Makarova soar into the air doing the splits or some such feat of physical prowess, be comforted that as long as you eat enough calcium and take enough exercise your bones will hold you up just as well as hers—and you won't even feel it!

AMATEUR ATHLETES, ALERT

"Anyone for tennis?" The sight of joggers, golfers, tennis players, and swimmers is a familiar one on the playgrounds of America. It's all good, healthy fun, of course, but a wise weekend sports enthusiast knows that there's more to a long, active, outdoor life than a summer workout.

"For people over college age who are not professional athletes, the most common sports injuries are muscle pulls, tendinitis, minor sprains and strains; what we call over-use syndromes," says orthopedic surgeon Dr. John L. Marshall, Director of Sports Medicine at New York's Hospital for Special Surgery. "And a lot of this has to do with the way people condition themselves to play. Unfortunately, most recreational athletes play to get in shape rather than get into shape to play. Thus they put demands on themselves which are beyond their physiological limits—not necessarily seriously so, but enough to cause them trouble and perhaps prevent them playing for a while."

Dr. Marshall is Orthopedic Consultant to the New York school system (seeing 4,500 children in contact sports), also to two Cornell University athletic teams and the U.S. ski team, and sees a variety of recreational and professional athletes—so he has seen a few injuries!

"The injuries come from excessive forces. These forces can result from moving too much one way, or moving the wrong way too much. An example: tennis elbow. Tennis elbow is brought on or aggravated by too much motion of the wrist, causing a muscle pull in the elbow. This gets accentuated by bad tennis, i.e., by the fact that you are whipping your wrist too much when you hit the ball. Weekend players make this mistake all the time. Thus, there is too much force repeatedly in one spot, causing tennis elbow."

Dr. Marshall mentions that a very stiff racket, whether steel or wood, will aggravate this condition. "It's the stiffness, plus the weight, that contributes to tennis elbow. A tennis racket should be light, with the right degree of flexibility, and strung properly, approximately 55 pounds."

A pulled leg muscle is caused by similar forces. "You have very tight structures in the back of your leg," explains Dr. Marshall, "making it hard to get your heel right down on the ground when you are moving around fast. If for some reason you jam your heel down when your muscle is contracted, you get a tear. In all these cases, what happens is that the muscle finally strains or fails."

LOOSE OR TIGHT-JOINTED?

A very useful discovery has recently been made in the field of sports injuries, which Dr. Marshall believes all amateur athletes should know about. "People may have loose or tight joints," he says, "and you should find out what you have, because they make you susceptible to different injuries. Loose-jointed people, for instance, are susceptible to kneecap trouble, because the kneecaps tend to drift and slide (Billie Jean King is an example). Such people may also be prone to dislocations and knee pain. Tight-jointed people are more susceptible to tendinitis of the elbow or shoulder, for instance. Also, these people suffer more muscle pulls and tears, pinched nerves, and back and neck problems.

"In football, where we have done a lot of research, we think we can predict with almost 80 percent accuracy, based on your body type, age, and exposure (i.e., level of competition), whether you are going to have a ligament or tendon injury. We need to do this in more sports—it is possible."

There are some simple tests to see if you are loose or tight—some you may have tried for fun as a child—for instance, seeing how far you can draw your thumb down (with your other hand) to touch your forearm, or, with wrist relaxed, how far you can bend your first finger back towards your forearm. A very loose-jointed person can lay his finger right down on the forearm. You can also be a mixture of both. One can have loose fingers, elbows, and shoulders, but be tight from pelvis to toes, for instance—a common case in women. According to Dr. Marshall, your looseness or tightness does not generally change with age. What changes is susceptibility as muscles become less flexible.

"Flexible muscles are very important," he says, "especially for the weekend athlete. You can play sports all you want on the weekend, but if you do nothing all week, your muscles will tighten up again and you'll be back where you started. That is why everyone should do flexibility exercises as a warm-up. One professional basketball player stopped flexibility exercises after doing them for years. The following season he was plagued by thigh muscle tears, ankle sprain, groin pull, and back pain. We used to go out and do calisthenics, but we now find that good flexibility is really what matters as far as preventing injuries is concerned."

Accidents will happen, however. Dr. Marshall sees them all the time. He has four instructions for sports enthusiasts who get a sprain or a pull. "*First*, rest. *Next*, make the muscle more flexible by doing stretching exercises. *Third*, make the muscle strong again with strengthening exercises. *Last*, find out what caused or aggravated the injury (a stiff racket, bad equipment, or wrong movements, for instance) so you can correct that. All those elements are essential for good treatment."

FOUR GUIDELINES FOR SPORTS FANS

1. Have a basic understanding of your capabilities. Know your own body type. This means evaluating what kind of an athlete you have been all your life—how you participated in school, college, and up to the present. This suggests a realistic approach to what *you* choose to do.

2. Get expert help. Talk to a coach or any professional in the discipline you have chosen. If you can, find a physician who

knows about sports to go over your history with you. But any good sports teacher can give you advice about a training program and learning the discipline of your sport.

3. Understand the sport you have chosen, so you start with some knowledge—what shoes to wear, what is the best equipment, and so forth. Read about the sport you want to play to keep up-to-date on conditioning, new ideas in the field—techniques, equipment.

4. Learn how to stretch your muscles properly with flexibility exercises that will minimize your susceptibility to injury. Do not strain; just stretch to the point where you feel an "easy" stretch. Hold the position without bouncing—then relax.

Chapter 5

LEGS AND FEET FIRST

"Her legs were long, slim, and shapely." That's the kind of novelist's line we can do without. The shape of legs, like feet and hands, is something you cannot alter much—except, of course, by keeping your weight down all over. But legs are more than art objects for other people's approval. They contain the strongest muscle in the body—the calf muscle— and they carry you about faithfully all your life, a job that is often neglected, or misunderstood.

DON'T CRAMP YOUR STYLE

Probably if you think of anything going wrong with your legs at all, you think of leg cramps. There are several causes for this pain, which can be very severe, according to Dr. Willibald Nagler, Chief of Physical Medicine and Rehabilitation at New York Hospital. "As one gets older, arterial problems can cause leg cramps, and these are often aggravated by smoking. You must remember that the arteries in the legs are very long—much longer than in the arms, for instance. They have to go all the way from the abdomen down to the ankles. In addition, the calf muscle has an extremely high demand for oxygen—it is a high-energy muscle—so blood circulation is very important. Smoking tends to contract the small blood vessels, inhibiting the flow of oxygen, thus producing cramps."

Dr. Nagler mentions two other causes of leg cramps: ill-fitting shoes (not just high heels), which force the calf muscles to do an extra balancing act; and too much loss of fluid, during excessive sweating, for example, as sometimes occurs with very energetic exercise.

OTHER ACHILLES HEELS

Leg cramps may feel bad: Swollen ankles look even worse. Swollen ankles are caused by an accumulation of fluid in the bottom of the legs. "Many women get an accumulation of fluid prior to menstruation," explains Dr. Nagler. "It's very natural, and it soon goes away. Another reason why you may get an accumulation of fluid in your ankles is because of weakened leg veins and muscles. If you stand for a very long time, the muscles cannot do their pumping action through veins, and fluid collects. Long sitting, such as on an airplane flight, can also cause this accumulation. (Varicose veins, too, which tend to be hereditary, can be triggered off by sitting or standing too long.)"

Basketball players are famous for their bad knees and pulled muscles. Luckily for us lesser mortals, our knees usually remain healthy unless we experience some form of osteoarthritis later in life, or unless we suddenly decide to start eating Japanese style. If you are overweight, however, you are much more likely to get stiff knees. There's too much stress on them. And if you do suddenly take it upon yourself to kneel down when you eat, take Dr. Nagler's advice: "Human nature hates sudden changes. In the West, we eat sitting down. Our knees are not used to more stress. Build them up slowly by bending and flexing them. Prepare them by kneeling down every day for a little while, increasing the time until you feel relaxed in that position."

If stiff knees aren't your Achilles heel, what is? The Achilles tendon is the tendon in the calf muscle that inserts into the heel. For normal walking about, it is absolutely necessary to have a healthy Achilles tendon. "When you walk, you press down first on the heel, then roll over and push off with the toes," says Dr. Nagler. "The Achilles tendon then contracts. It must be prepared for this. If you do some forceful activity suddenly, like skiing or playing tennis, and the tendon is not prepared, then you can rupture it."

A pulled muscle is caused by similar forces. The tight muscles in the back of the leg can be stretched too hard if you jam your heel down while running, skiing, or reaching for a ball, for instance. If you do this when the muscle is contracted, then you'll get a tear.

GIVE YOUR LEGS A LIFT

For healthy legs and ankles, some basic rules of nurture are offered by Dr. Nagler:

1. Do some stretching exercises every day to avoid muscle or tendon pulls and joint stiffness (very important if you wish to exercise).

2. For walking, wear low heels. At all times, wear shoes that fit snugly round the heel and loosely enough round the toes for them to wiggle. "Choose leather or fabric that allows your feet to breathe and be flexible," adds podiatrist Dr. Roberts. "Soles should be leather or crepe rubber—as long as they are flexible." For more on shoes, see p. 329.

3. Keep your legs moving to prevent accumulation of fluid in the ankles. If you have to stand or sit for long periods, run in place or move from one foot to the other as much as possible to allow the veins and muscles to do their work.

4. Wear support hose if you have a tendency to varicose veins or have to stand for long periods. For this to be effective, the pressure should be strongest around the ankle and decrease as it goes up the calf. This pressure stimulates fluid dynamics, preventing accumulation.

5. Try putting your legs up for 10 to 15 minutes a day, in a position higher than your head, to drain excess fluid out of the legs.

FOOT-LOOSE AND FANCY-FREE

Sounds lovely, doesn't it? The interesting thing is that being fancy-free has a lot more to do with your feet than you might imagine. Unhappy feet, whether through bad circulation, aching muscles, poor balance, or constricting shoes, can cause backache, neck pain, and an allover feeling of fatigue. (Young people, particularly, who complain of tiredness and lack of energy are often found simply to be wearing the wrong kind of shoes.)

Americans are, however, becoming much more foot-conscious—particularly women. According to Dr. Nathaniel Gould, former Chief Orthopedic Surgeon at Brockton Hospital, Massachusetts, and a founder and former president of the American Orthopaedic Foot Society, Inc., most women today are wearing shoes that are practical and comfortable. "As far back as the fourteenth century," he says, "we find high heels and pointed toes for women. People in the past paid no attention to comfort. But today with women out of the house, doing jobs that men were doing, they are on their feet much more and find it's essential to be comfortable."

There are new developments afoot in orthopedics, too, Dr. Gould points out. The American Orthopaedic Foot Society, founded only six years ago for research and education into foot problems, works closely with shoe manufacturers in trying to produce better-shaped shoes. One of its earliest successes was getting manufacturers to stop making pointed-toed shoes for children, in vogue at the time. A big effort is being made to "educate the man in the shoe store" to give you the right design and fit. "I can see the time," says Dr. Gould, "when you will walk into a shoe store in the morning; casts will be made of your feet; and you will return in the afternoon to pick up your shoes."

There is also exciting news for the feet of the future. "We have discovered that certain defects of the feet (for example, calcaneo-vulgus feet, where the feet muscles and ligaments have been stretched, causing painful and inhibiting flat feet) are a predisposition before birth and can be diagnosed at that time. This means a baby can be given corrective surgery within the first six months, which is when it is most effective. Before now, flat feet sufferers had little recourse. Children today can start out with healthy feet and straight legs," says Dr. Gould.

FIVE FANCY-FREE FOOT CARE TIPS

1. Take care of your feet as much as you take care of your hands—wash them; cream them; trim the nails (straight across, which helps prevent ingrowing toenails); keep them clean.

2. Walk a little more. The chief way that blood comes uphill from the lower extremities is by action of the muscles on the veins. If the muscles are not exercised steadily every day to some degree, they tend to get stasis of the circulation and a tiredness, which affects you all over. Circulation is improved just by motion—you don't have to climb or jog, just walk at your own most comfortable pace.

3. Do foot exercises (for instance, walking on the ball of the foot) and massage the feet to help circulation and take out some of the tiredness. Circulation of the feet has really to be worked on since the feet are so far away from the heart. When you are resting and put your feet up, put them not just off the floor but higher than your heart.

4. Watch out for callouses and corns. They mean something is wrong. Corns are usually attributed to confining footwear. Callouses mean there is something wrong with the way you are standing or walking or in the way your feet hit the floor. Your shock absorbers aren't working properly, creating hard

skin. See your doctor for either of these problems—they can be corrected.

5. Wear the right shoes. This is a huge subject, but briefly, follow these guidelines:

   a. Wear leather soles and shoes. Leather is soft, flexible, and allows the foot to breathe. Rubber heels are fine and prevent skidding, but thick rubber soles are not good for long periods of time—they disturb the breathability of the foot, so it will perspire and get tired.

   b. Shoes should be as light as possible. Think how many times you pick up your feet—the added weight of the shoe only creates more effort.

   c. Wear boots only for protection against the elements or for sports or certain jobs. They can be very tiring.

   d. Wear as low heels as possible. High heels throw you off balance. To see what this means, strip down in front of a long mirror and watch yourself walk across the room in high heels. The knee has to be bent; the hip also bends; the lumbar region has to make an extra high arch; the neck cranes; the head is held badly. The higher the heel, the more you curve. As a matter of fact, if you are wearing a 2-inch heel you do not automatically become 2 inches taller, because your body is having to make these compensatory curves for balance. High heels also thwart the motion of the foot from going through its shock-absorbing action, which affects the joints all the way up the leg and into your back and up to your neck, jarring your whole body.

The act of wearing shoes is not what's wrong—it's wearing shoes not proper for *you.* Have a foot checkup to find out the predispositions of your feet with an orthopedic surgeon specializing in feet, or at a foot clinic (these are now being set up all over the country in response to this new foot-consciousness). Then you can find the right shoes for you. For instance, when you try it on, you should measure the width of the shoe sole to make certain it is big enough and learn how high your arch is—a person with a high arch should have a shoe that fits the arch and supports it. Lower arches need similarly lower-arched shoes. Wiggle your toes in the shoe—the "toe box" should be deep enough not to press your toes. See that the shoe has a straight inside last—so that your inside heel and big toe are in a straight line.

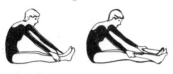

HAMSTRING STRETCH (BACK OF THIGH)

Sit down with your legs straight, heels no more than 6 inches apart. Reach down and get an easy stretch. You will probably feel it in the back of your thighs. If you have trouble stretching and simultaneously relaxing in this position, use a towel to help. Put the towel around your feet, grab the ends, and pull yourself forward to where you can relax and stretch. Work your way down the towel until you feel sufficiently stretched.

HAMSTRING STRETCH USING WALL

Choose an object near you such as a wall, tree, or table, or anything which is about waist high or at a height from which you can comfortably stretch. Place the back of your heel on the object, keeping your leg straight out. Your leg on the ground should be nearly straight (people with back problems should bend the knee slightly), with your foot pointed

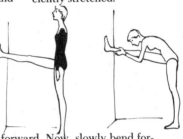

forward. Now, slowly bend forward at the waist until you feel a good stretch in the back of the raised leg. Hold this position, then relax.

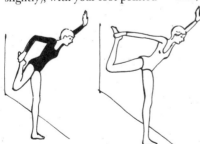

QUADRICEPS STRENGTH (FRONT OF THIGH)

Stand on one foot. Hold on to the wall with your left hand. Stand far enough away from it so that your left arm is kept fairly straight. Reach behind you and grab your right foot from the outside with your right hand. Now slowly pull your foot toward your buttocks until you feel the stretch in the front of your thigh. Hold this stretch for 15-25 seconds. For a greater stretch, hold the same position, then slowly extend your leg backward into your right hand, intensifying the stretch on your thigh (right picture). This will straighten out your left arm.

CALF STRETCHES

Face a wall, standing about 2 feet away from it. Rest your forearms on the wall with your forehead on the back of your hands. Now bend one knee and bring that knee toward the wall. Keep your other leg straight and the heel down as you move your hips slightly toward the wall. Keep your toes pointed straight ahead. (Left picture.) You should feel a good stretch in the calf of the left leg. If you want to stretch the Achilles' tendon from this position, slightly bend the back knee, keeping the foot flat (right picture). This gives you a much lower stretch, which is also good for maintaining or regaining ankle flexibility. By stretching one leg at a time as described, you are able to isolate and control the stretch in the calf muscle.

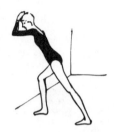 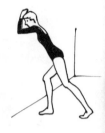

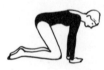

QUADRICEPS AND KNEE STRETCH

First kneel down, placing your hands on the outside of your ankles. Walk backward with your hands so that they are behind you. Place your hands as far back as you can. Hold and feel the stretch on the front of your ankles, shins, and thighs. CAUTION: If you have or have had knee problems, be very careful bending the knees behind you. Do it slowly and under control.

Chapter 6

BEAUTY FROM THE NECK UP

Once upon a time, in Japan, the nape of a woman's neck was considered erotic. Customs have changed in Japan (gone are those piled-up, lacquered, neck-exposing hairstyles, for one thing). But in America, where nobody ever paid much attention to napes of necks, things are pretty much the same. We still overlook the neck—not just the nape, but the whole thing. Until something goes wrong. It is no accident that spoiled children and leaky faucets, among other aggravating things, are *not* called "a pain in the ankle." Neck ailments of varying severity are right up there with headaches as one of our nation's leading . . . well, pains in the neck (in matters of health, anyway).

A PAIN IN THE NECK

Dr. Bernard Jacobs, Clinical Professor of Orthopedic Surgery at Cornell University, modestly describes neck problems as "very common." But the fact that at New York's Hospital for Special Surgery there is a whole clinic for neck problems (Dr. Jacobs heads this clinic) speaks for itself. "I call the neck the Times Square of the human frame," says Dr. Jacobs. "The spinal cord goes through it, and all the nerves to the arm and the two main arteries to the brain. All of these can be affected by neck disorders." So when neck pain is accompanied by nerve symptoms (pain, numbness, or a pins-

and-needles feeling in your extremities) or frequent head-aches or dizziness, you should see an orthopedist. These symptoms could indicate joint or disk problems, which can be treated a number of ways—with exercises, collars to relieve stress, heat packs traction, and certain drugs.

For all neck discomfort, from that stiffness that the English call "desk neck" (the result of sitting at a desk in a high-tension environment) to trauma-related problems (often, an incipient disc or joint problem is discovered only after provocation by some kind of accident), Dr. Jacobs recommends these measures for easing the neck's burden: (1) If you must bend down, don't bend from the waist (the neck goes down); squat, bending the knees. (2) Avoid reaching for things on top shelves (in other words, don't stretch your arms above your head too strenuously). (3) Avoid turning your head quickly (if, for instance, someone calls you). Use the rearview mirror when driving, instead of craning your neck around to see what's behind you. (4) If you play tennis, don't stretch your arm too far bac ∶ or up when serving; you may have to modify your serve to achieve this. (5) If you do a lot of gardening, do your pruning, etc., while sitting on a stool, to avoid bending your neck down while stooping. Dr. Jacobs has many gardeners among his patients. For tension-relieving exercises, Dr. Jacobs is fond of "shoulder shrugs." "Shrug your shoulders," he says, "and hold them shrugged to a count of 3. Then relax. Do this 20 times." He also has some isometric techniques: Put one hand behind the head and push the head back against it (without letting the hand yield)—slowly, and without tension. Hold this position to a count of 3, then relax. Repeat the process with the hand on the forehead and the head pressing forward. Then do it with the hand on the right side of the head, and finally, on the left side of the head. Do the push-release routine 20 times in each direction.

"Massage," says Dr. Jacobs, "is useful, but only as a temporary thing." He recommends it as a warm-up before and after doing the exercises. First, apply a heat pack.

(Commercially made packs, wet or dry, are available at drugstores and surgical appliance stores.) Then massage your neck. "It's better," Dr. Jacobs suggests, "if you have somebody you like do it for you." Do the exercises and afterwards, apply more heat and have another massage. If all this seems like too much trouble, you can get heat and massage simultaneously by doing shoulder shrugs under a warm, strong shower.

THE TELLTALE THROAT

A neck problem which is not merely common but universal, and which may not be physically painful but causes great unhappiness, is the crepey neck that comes with the creeping-on of years. "Most women forget for years that they have a neck," says New York skin expert Mario Badescu. "But the skin on the neck is very thin and sensitive, and the first signs of old age appear here, the wrinkles and the folding." The aging process, however, is not the only reason for lines. Imperfect posture, or any activity in which the neck is bent frequently (writing, talking on the telephone, crocheting), can cause the neck skin to "age" before its time.

Badescu recommends light massage to help straighten out the problem. "Apply a little cream on the neck," he says, "and use a tapping movement toward the back of the neck, following the lines drawn by folds of skin in the neck. Massage very slowly, and not hard. Just touch the skin." Lying as flat as possible when sleeping in bed (in other words, no fat pillows, or no pillow at all), is also helpful.

Walking around with a book on your head helps to correct that line-etching slump. Badescu also suggests the following "neck roll" exercise as a great skin-smoother and muscle-loosener. Sit on the floor, "lotus" or "Indian" style. Drop the head forward—*gently.* Inhale, rolling the head clockwise (keep your shoulder *down;* the tendency is to raise it slightly to "meet" the head), then back. Exhale, continuing the head movement over the left shoulder, bringing the head back to its original position, facing front, lowered. The whole circle should be inscribed smoothly, in one continuous motion. Repeat it 10 times. Then circle the head counterclockwise ten times. For a double chin: Hold your head all the way back, stick your chin forward, and move your jaw gently from right to left ten times. Another useful chin exercise: Hold your head back and make a chewing motion up and down.

In addition to proper exercise, necks need moisture. "The neck should be cleaned twice a day, just like the face," says Badescu. "Use tepid water, never hot or cold, and avoid strong soap because it removes the acid mantle of the neck, making it very hard to maintain its youthfulness. And don't forget moisturizer, no matter what kind of skin you have." Also, since alcohol has drying properties, never spray cologne or use alcohol-based lotions on the neck. They remove the natural moisture from the skin. When you use a masque on your face, extend the treatment to the neck. Egg-yolk-and-oil or milk-and-honey masques are particularly good.

New York skin and beauty expert Janet Sartin does not believe in neck massage. She suggests the following pampering treatment. Cleanse the neck with a rich cleansing oil, the richest you can find. Apply an extra heavy night cream on the area. Take a thin layer of cotton just short of your neck size; saturate half of it with a rich moisturizing oil and fold the other half over it. Stretch the cotton over the neck surface fairly tightly. Lie down for 10–15 minutes. This is also a good treatment for the under-eye area (but don't use the treatment on blemished skin).

Dr. Stephen Kurtin, Assistant Clinical Professor of Dermatology at Mt. Sinai School of Medicine, agrees that the neck needs lots of moisturizer, either in cream or lotion form (the only difference between them is that creams are heavier). "What gives the skin moisture," says Dr. Kurtin, "is the amount of water in the skin. So apply moisturizer when your skin is still slightly damp. Oils don't give you moisture: They help to retain the moisture content of the skin."

Although from Dr. Jacobs's point of view, one of the neck's worst enemies is gardening, Dr. Kurtin sees things in another light—sunlight, to be exact. The sun is the *skin's* worst enemy, and, as has been mentioned, neck skin is particularly delicate. "A lot of my patients are models," says Dr. Kurtin, "and if you get a wrinkle, you may be unhappy. But if they get wrinkles, they may be out of a job. In the summer, you see these models walking around in hats, not for fashion but to keep the sun off their faces." And necks. Clothes, of course, are the best protection. But if you must be in the sun, or can't subscribe to the newborn fashion dictum, "Pale is beautiful," do use sunblocking or sun-sceening preparations. Dr. Kurtin likes any product with PABA, which allows tanning but prevents burning. And only sunbathe before 11 A.M. and after 3 P.M.

The one thing that can be said of all these neck-saving measures is that, although there is no known prevention for age, its effects can be minimized. And the sooner you begin, the better. (See exercises, below and p. 70).

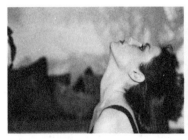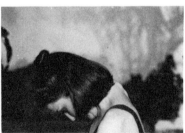

To correct a double chin, drop head back, stick chin straight out, move jaw gently right to left 10 times. Then drop head down.

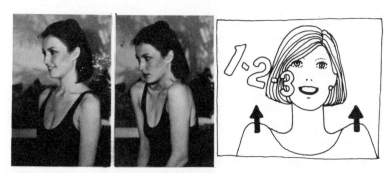

Shoulder shrugs are recommended by orthopedist Dr. Bernard Jacobs as a way to relieve neck tension. Shrug shoulders, hold to a count of 3, relax. Repeat 20 times.

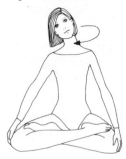

Neck-roll exercise is a good muscle loosener, tension-easer. Drop head forward, gently inhale, and roll head clockwise, keeping shoulders down; exhale. Then roll head slowly in the other direction, until it is back in original position, lowered.

LEND ME YOUR EARS

The joy of music, the voice of someone you love, the sound of a bird singing, or silence—pleasures granted us by that most remarkable of instruments, the human ear. Not only does the ear allow us to hear what goes on in the world, but it also works to keep us on our feet.

It consists of three parts. The outer ear is the part you see—a shell-like cartilage with many folds to catch the sound waves. It is covered by skin, which very closely adheres to this underlying cartilage. This is important, because if you get even a tiny ear infection, there is very little room for swelling, and the pain is therefore much greater than you would expect. The cartilage of this outer ear continues along a canal until it meets part of the mastoid bone, which goes to the eardrum—a distance of roughly 1 to 1½ inches. This canal is lined with fine hairs and some 2,000 wax producing glands. Since it is covered with skin, it also contains sweat and sebaceous glands. The job of the outer ear is to gather sounds from the air and pass them on to the eardrum, which vibrates. These vibrations are then conducted into the inner ear, the organ of hearing.

The middle ear, on the other side of the eardrum, has three tiny bones (the smallest bones in your body) which conduct the eardrum's vibrations to the inner ear. The inner ear contains two very delicate organs, housed in the mastoid bone (the hardest bone in your body)—the cochlea, which is shaped like a shell, and three small chambers, which control your balance. The cochlea contains the organ of Corti, which is covered with many fine hairs arranged like the strings on a harp. Here the vibrations of sound are changed into nerve impulses and conducted to the hearing center of the brain. The organ of balance contains semicircular canals, filled with fluid, monitoring your sense of balance. If you close your eyes and tilt your head, you can feel it—because the fluid in these canals has tipped. Seasickness is the result of the malfunctioning of the semicircular canals—when rapid, irregular, and continuous waves of motion persist, your balance is disturbed.

By the age of ten, your hearing is at its keenest—as many as 20,000 vibrations per second. By thirty, it's down to about 15,000. As you get older, your blood supply diminishes, and since the two organs of the inner ear are supplied by only one blood vessel, obviously hearing is affected—it's simply part of the aging process.

There are, however, ways you can keep your ears at their finely tuned best, according to Dr. S. Evans Ganz, Attending Surgeon, Manhattan Eye, Ear, and Throat Hospital, and Diplomate of the American Board of Otolaryngology. Here are his suggestions:

1. Clean your ears with a washcloth only. Wax is a protec-

tive mechanism in the ear that nature provided, and normally it loosens itself and falls out. Pushing cotton-tipped sticks or other things in the ear to dislodge wax simply pushes the wax further down the canal into the eardrum where it cannot possibly escape and affects your hearing. If you do have a problem with wax (some people simply have more active wax glands than others) have it professionally removed. "In fact," says Dr. Ganz, "I don't advise putting anything down the ear—sticks, drops, fingers—they can all cause infection. The old adage that you shouldn't put anything smaller than your elbow in your ear makes excellent sense."

2. Protect your ears against extreme cold or heat. "Since the skin of the ear adheres very closely to the underlying cartilage," explains Dr. Ganz, "and since blood supply to the ear is not profuse, the ear is highly subject to changes in temperature, particularly to frostbite. Both frostbite and severe burns come from the same cause, a disturbance of the blood supply tissues. All skiers should cover their ears."

3. If you have a cold, do not fly. If you must fly for reasons of emergency, spray your nose with a nasal spray. "This is very important," Dr. Ganz says. "When you have a cold, your nose is congested, and the pressure spreads from the nose along the eustachian tubes to the ears. If you fly, what happens? No plane is completely pressurized—so there is increased pressure in your ears. With a cold, that double pressure can rupture your eardrum. And the precaution is so simple—if only more people knew about it—a nasal spray opens the tubes and prevents that pressure. In fact, it's not a bad idea to do it even if you haven't got a cold. This also holds true with scuba diving—if you have a cold, use the spray before you dive."

4. Avoid loud noises if possible. Children who listen to very loud pop music constantly are damaging their hearing nerve

and will be hard of hearing at an early age. Industrial noise causes the same damage. Anyone exposed to excessive noise should wear earmuffs or earplugs as long as they are not of a very hard material—this is the only exception to the "nothing in the ear" rule.

To know more about your ears is, perhaps, to appreciate them more—and to care for them means that you can continue to be enchanted, in Shakespeare's words, by the "noises, sounds, and sweet airs, that give delight."

Chapter 7

PUTTING YOUR BEST FACE FORWARD

The human face is a fascinating thing. It can speak volumes. It can inspire poetry. It can launch a thousand ships. We may forget a name, but we rarely forget a face. "We have," says Desmond Morris in *The Naked Ape*, "the most subtle and complex facial expression system of all living animals. By making tiny movements of the flesh around the mouth, nose, eyes, eyebrows, and on the forehead, and by recombining the movements in a wide variety of ways, we can convey a whole range of complex mood-changes." It is hardly surprising, then, that the look of our faces should play such an enormous part in our lives. Right from its first wrinkled, bumpy, pink appearance on this earth, the face is in the limelight.

But it's the skin that people care about—a smooth, youthful, dewy-fresh skin for ever and ever. The things that have been written about skin care could probably fill several branches of a public library. Nobody knows more about the subject than the two doctors consulted here: Each one has chosen to speak about an area of skin that concerns him. Each piece of advice they give can give your skin a new lease on life—and that means *now*.

FOUR VITAL QUESTIONS ABOUT YOUR SKIN

Dr. Samuel M. Peck, Professor of Dermatology Emeritus, Mount Sinai School of Medicine, New York City:

What helps dry skin?

Moisture is given off by the skin in two forms: (1) by insensible perspiration, which is the moisture that is put on the surface of your skin from your sweat (so sweat is a good moisturizer); and (2) by the slow loss of water given out, not through the sweat glands, but through all the layers of the skin from the blood stream and from the skin itself.

Dry skin in an otherwise normal, healthy person, is due to the fact that the upper layers of the skin, which are dead, do not retain the natural moisture as long as they are meant to. Most often this is due to a dry atmosphere—in parts of the country such as the Southwest, or in overheated rooms anywhere. Also some people lack certain substances in these upper layers of skin (keratin), which help bind water to the skin.

Now if you took the top layer of dead skin, or keratin, from your body, as an experiment, and put it in a dehydrator to take out the moisture, it would look like a piece of leather, dry and brittle. You try to bend it and it snaps. But if you put that "leather" in water it at once becomes soft and pliable again. If, on the other hand, you cover the dehydrated keratin with all the grease in the world, from mineral grease to the finest lanolin, it will still be as stiff as a board. In other words, dryness of the skin has nothing to do with lack of oiliness—it is simply a question of water.

Modern moisturizers put moisture back in the skin because they are formulated so that the skin will take up water from the cream, and the cream won't fight the skin for water. Another way of moisturizing is to use petroleum jelly, which moisturizes the skin by a different method. It acts as a barrier so water can't get out, and you moisturize yourself.

Glycerine and rosewater were once considered to be fine treatment for dry skin. We now know that glycerine has a very peculiar property—it absorbs water. So if glycerine were used on the skin on its own, it would tend to dry it. However, glycerine is put into some cosmetics in order to keep them from drying out, but they are formulated not to dry your skin. The very effective modern moisturizers are water-and-oil emulsions.

How does diet affect your skin?

It is important that you discuss diet with your own doctor to find out what is best for your skin. The average known standards of vitamins and adequate nutrition do very well for a normal skin. But some of us have a different metabolism and have different absorption not only of vitamins but of other components of the diet as well. Let us take an example: There are some individuals, usually in the age group between about twenty and forty, who develop very dry skin, and in addition, the skin has what we call keratoses, that is, little gatherings of dry skin above the surface. In mild cases, they are often seen on the upper thighs and upper arms; in extreme cases, on the forehead, chest, and even hands.

The reason is this: These people have an inherited characteristic called dysvitaminosis A, where the normal amount of vitamin A in their foods is either not absorbed adequately or is not utilized properly in the body. So they need extremely large doses (as much as 100,000 units a day or more) to have a relatively normal skin.

Some people claim that enormous doses of vitamin A will prevent blackheads (apart from those suffering from dysvitaminosis A). Within limits, this is true. But the amount needed by mouth is so large that it is unwarranted, in view of the possible side effects (loss of hair, skin eruptions). However, there has been a tremendous discovery very recently that sidetracks or avoids the excessive use of vitamin A. It is now possible to isolate vitamin A acid, and this acid, used in a cream, with judicious application, *decreases black-heads and may, in fact, actually cure them.* The name of the cream is Retin A cream, made by Johnson & Johnson, available by prescription only.

An important way diet affects skin is in the case of acne. An excess of iodine in the diet, while it is not the cause of acne (usually a hormonal disturbance plus bacteria), very often makes the acne worse—depending on which part of the country you live in. If you live at the seaboard, there is less tendency to need iodine than there is in the Middle West. I've tried to make iodized salt, for instance, illegal in the states that do not need it. Iodized salt, and foods like shrimp, oysters, and clams, contain enough iodine to aggravate a case of acne.

How do you recognize skin cancer?

In our affluent society, large segments of our population do not give their skin a rest period, but worship the sun all year round. That is why I think skin cancer due to actinic damage (caused by excessive sunlight) is on the increase. And if you are a redhead, or have freckles, then you are also more prone to sun exposure and skin cancers than other people.

If you have a small scaly tumor (little growth) that looks like a wart but is not in the place a wart would normally be, such as the feet or hands; and if it grows, and if it bleeds, then you should instantly consult your doctor or dermatologist. In older people, about fifty, a common skin cancer called basal cell cancer manifests itself as a small ulcer that doesn't heal. Again, consult your doctor. These cancers, which are about 90 percent of the cancers we see, are curable in more than 95 percent of cases.

More serious skin cancers are much larger ulcers, and it is not likely that you would neglect them. The final group are the cancers that arise from moles. Now there are many people walking around with moles who are perfectly healthy. The average mole rarely turns into a cancer. However, if one of those moles becomes very black, gets bigger, and especially if it tends to bleed or become inflamed, please consult an authority. (During pregnancy, moles tend to grow a little, so don't be alarmed.) Another recent discovery is that certain moles develop a halo around them, that is, a ring around them that has no pigment. If you notice this consult a doctor. Any lumps, either on or under the skin, that do not disappear, especially on the breasts, should be reported at once.

What is the pH factor?

PH is the measurement of the acid-alkaline balance of your skin, and it is a very important factor in healthy skin.

Some years ago, I did some research into the content of sweat in order to discover if it bore any relationship to the localization of skin diseases. We were able to show that sweat contains elements, fatty acids, that protect the skin against infection.

These protective agents fight infection best when your skin is at its normal pH measurement—below 7—which is a little on the acid side (7 is neutral; above 7 is alkaline). The environment (sun, wind, chlorinated water, alkaline soaps, and so forth) tends to make the skin more alkaline, but preparations you use can bring it back to its normal, healthiest pH. For instance, if you wash your hair with an alkaline shampoo, use a rinse that will balance it, or if you wash your face with an alkaline soap, follow it with a preparation (moisturizer, lotion, makeup) that will balance it. (Also, some products are labeled "acid balanced" or "non-alkaline." Or you can test any product by dipping into it Nitrazine papers, litmuslike papers; you can get them at your pharmacy.)

SEVEN WAYS TO CARE FOR YOUR SKIN

Dr. Albert M. Kligman, Professor of Dermatology at the University of Pennsylvania School of Medicine:

1. Clean your face with mild soap, cleansing milks, or creams *in moderation.* Twice a day should be enough. Your face is cleaner than you think. Too much cleaning over the years can cause damage.

2. Occasional mild massage with a gently abrasive cloth or cold water stimulates the blood flow in facial skin and helps it to look its best.

3. Keep the surface of your skin smooth with emollients—most moisturizers and creams do the job. Emollients will keep the skin's surface in its best condition, but will not retard the aging process. What happens in aging skin is that the fibrous substance of the skin itself deteriorates, mainly through exposure to sunlight, and the cells, which normally come off one at a time, come off in big clumps, so that the skin can look dry and scaly. Moisturizers and creams can smooth the outside surface of the skin and reduce friction (particularly important in winter and when resting the face against pillows at night).

4. Keep your face as protected as possible from sunlight. Wear hats and use protective creams. Too much sun causes wrinkling and fine lines.

5. Keep your hands away from your face as much as possible, to avoid wrinkling the skin and further irritating any blemishes you may have. Remember this when watching television, working at a desk, or reading. Continual changes in expression can cause wrinkling, too, particularly around the eyes, when the skin is expanding and contracting thousands of times a day. If you were never to smile, never get angry, never grimace, never laugh, *and* stay in the dark, your skin would stay as smooth as a child's—but what kind of a person would you be if you lived like that?

6. Keep the temperature of the rooms in your house *down* and the humidity *high.* This is particularly important, of course, in winter. The lower the thermostat, the better for

your complexion. It's good for your furniture and the energy crisis, too!

7. Blackheads and pimples should be allowed to grow out by themselves normally or be removed professionally. Do not attempt to remove them yourself, as they can cause scars.

A blackhead is an accretion that does not leave the follicle, a filling in of the canal with fibrous protein. Ask your doctor for advice if blackheads are a problem for you.

YOUNG SKIN FOREVER?

Nobody's worked a miracle—yet. A seventy-year-old woman isn't suddenly going to look twenty. But there's something very definitely in the air. "We have been using vitamin A acid (Retin A cream) to try to restore some of the damage which takes place in aging skin," says Dr. Kligman. "It's a very unusual drug. We have been using it with some success for acne, but we now know it has multiple effects in the treatment of aging skin:

1. The surface of the skin is made smoother. If someone is very wrinkled and the skin is very loose, obviously vitamin A acid is not going to tighten up the face. The laxity of old skin is there forever. But the drug can reduce scaliness in a controlled fashion, and it is safer than operations such as dermabrasion or phenol chemosurgery.

2. Pigmentation diminishes. As you get older, the skin on face and hands tends to mottle. Vitamin A acid reduces that blotchy appearance.

3. It cleans out the follicles. With age, your skin follicles get larger, and they fill up with tiny little hairs too small to see. If a woman of fifty or sixty complains that her complexion is getting coarser, it is because the follicles, which used to contain one hair, now contain from 5 to 30 hairs. Vitamin A acid has the tendency to expel those hair plugs—that alone improves the look of the skin.

4. The fibrous tissue is improved. In sun-damaged skin, for instance, elastic fibrous tissue is laid down beneath the epidermis in excessive amounts—it is like leather, quite insoluble and stable. Vitamin A acid removes that abnormal deposition of elastic fiber, and we hope it may be replaced by newer, fresher tissue.

5. It stimulates the epidermis. We think vitamin A acid puffs up the top layer of the skin a little bit, thus making it look fuller and smoother.

6. It has an anti-tumor effect. Skin lesions or tumors, especially on the back of the hand, can be treated, and their appearance retarded, by vitamin A acid.

Exciting? Dr. Kligman thinks so, but he emphasizes that its use for aging skin is still in the experimental stage. "Our next stage is to learn how to use it," he explains. "Up to now, we may have been too conservative. It has side effects, too. It produces redness and irritation, so you have to be prepared for that. But if it is used generously and enthusiastically, as kids with acne tend to use it, it may pay off. At the moment, the concentrations we are using are entirely empirical. We are just putting it on and watching. This is a preliminary report."

A preliminary report—but in spite of his caution, Dr. Kligman believes that if regarded in a sensible way, this drug may obtain cosmetically useful results even if it is not a restoration to youth. What a present to American skin!

Chapter 8

TAKE A PAIR OF SPARKLING EYES

They say you can tell a person by his eyes. They say the eye is the window of the soul. They say your eyes are the only part of you that never grows old. Superstitions about eyes are commonplace—yet how much do we really know about them?

EYEBALL TO EYEBALL

"The human eye is made up of a variety of tissues, some transparent, and some opaque," explains Dr. A. Benedict Rizzuti, Consultant Ophthalmologist, New York Eye and Ear Infirmary and Methodist Hospital of Brooklyn, Clinical Professor of Ophthalmology at New York Medical College, and board member of the International Eye Foundation and the Better Vision Institute.

"Let us start with the outside of the eye," he says, "the upper and lower lids, which protect the whole mechanism. Then we have the window of the eye, which is known as the cornea. Behind the cornea is an optically empty space, after which comes the iris, which constricts the light like the diaphragm of a camera, and which will dilate in the dark. In the center of the iris is an opening, called the pupil, which appears black. Behind the iris is the lens—which takes its name from the word "lentil," because that is what it looks like. The lens is transparent and allows light rays to pass through and converge on the back of the eye, known as the retina. The retina can be compared to the film of a camera, which takes the picture. Sensation is carried from the retina, follows along the path of the optic nerve, which is on the back part of the eye, and relayed to the brain.

"Many people ask, what is *inside* the eye? Two elements— one is a fluid, known as the aqueous, meaning that it is like water. This is located in the space between the cornea and the front surface of the iris and is the plumbing system of the eye. Behind the iris and lens we have the other element; that fills the globe. This is called the vitreous—a jellylike mass, which has practically no function except to hold all tissues in their normal relationship, giving the globe the correct outline and tension."

The eye, evidently, is a complex mechanism. But there is one thing the human eye lacks that the lower animals possess—a neurilemma sheath, or protective covering of the optic nerve. "The reason why this is important," says Dr. Rizzuti, "is that in fish, for example, you can transplant a whole eye, and it will take. In humans, because there is no neurilemma sheath to heal or knit together the cut ends of the optic nerves, you cannot transplant the whole eye successfully. You can only transplant a part of the eye, like the cornea."

According to Dr. Rizzuti, most people are born slightly farsighted, and there are many more farsighted people in the world than nearsighted. (Most animals, dogs, for instance, are also farsighted.) But as we get older, that far sight gradually tends toward near sight. The cornea and the lens begin to get hazy; the jelly of the eye breaks down; and we get changes in the retina. The human eye, it seems, is not a perfect machine.

EYES AND NOES

There are ways to care for our eyes so that even this

imperfect machine can last and look beautiful longer. Dr. Rizzuti suggests the following advice for people with normal, healthy eyes:

1. Protect your eyes with glasses from unusual hazards such as work around machinery, dusty atmospheres, fumes or chemicals. (In industry, protective goggles are mandatory in hazardous occupations.) A highly chlorinated pool, for instance, can irritate eyes. If you swim a lot, use goggles. Copious washing of the eyes with water is the best emergency therapy for chemical burns of the eyes.

2. Wear sunglasses in the sun and snow. Too bright light can burn the retina. Wearing sunglasses as a routine procedure, however, indoors all day and all night, is not so wise. You become dependent—as soon as you take the glasses off, you may get a sensitivity of the eye known as photophobia, in which the eye will start to water and smart. So wear sunglasses when exposed to sun or snow—not all the time. Do not wear sunglasses for night driving for they cut down on your vision considerably.

   (If you wear glasses and are very aware of light refracting through the glass, you may be hypersensitive to light. In this situation, you may require a pink or preferably green tint in your lenses—but the tint should not be dark.)

3. Wash your eyes in moderation only. Nature gives us certain fluids to lubricate the eyes (tears, for instance, are a natural fluid and act as a lubricant) producing a protective coating for the cornea. We should not disturb that fluid by excessive washing.

4. Dry skin around the eyes or eyelids may be caused by an allergy. Allergic reactions are individual responses to a source of irritation, and your own experience is the best detective in these cases.

5. Take mascara or eyeliner off as thoroughly as possible every night. Too much mascara worn over a number of years

can leave a deposit on the inner lining of the eyelid and cause irritation. If your eyes continually itch or become red when you are wearing eye makeup, it could be an allergy, so see your doctor.

6. Cold compresses can be very soothing to inflamed eyes. If your eyes are exposed to too much sun or are otherwise inflamed, a solution of half witch hazel and half cold water, or cold water on its own, soothes and relieves the inflammation.

7. Read in a good light. Bad light can cause eye fatigue, eye strain, and headaches. The best light for reading is a combination of incandescent light (table or standard lamps) and fluorescent overhead lighting. Fluorescent lighting as direct light on its own is often fatiguing.

8. Lots of sleep is good for eyes. Lack of sleep causes a congestion of the tissues and redness. Also drinking too much alcohol can abnormally dilate the blood vessels. (Some people with very superficial blood vessels in their eyes can get redness from wind or everyday dust, but this is not usual.) If you continue to have red eyes, see your doctor.

9. Healthy eyes need a good balanced diet. Some of the eye problems in underdeveloped countries, where Dr. Rizzuti frequently travels and works, are due to poor diet, particularly vitamin A deficiency and lack of protein.

10. Have regular checkups, particularly as you get older. At forty, certain physiological changes take place in the eye. One normal symptom is difficulty in reading very fine print at close range—and if that is so, you may need reading glasses. Also at forty, Dr. Rizzuti urges that *every* individual have the pressure taken of his or her eyes, so that an underlying glaucoma condition, which tends to creep up on a person at that time, may be spotted and treated good and early.

MINI EYE QUIZ

Q. What's the difference between an ophthalmologist, an oculist, an optometrist, and an optician?
A. An ophthalmologist or oculist is a physician—an M.D.— who specializes in diagnosis and treatment of defects and diseases of the eye, performing surgery if necessary. An optometrist is a licensed, nonmedical practitioner who measures refractive errors—that is, irregularities in the size or shape of the eyeball or surface of the cornea—and eye muscle disturbances. In his treatment, the optometrist uses glasses, prisms, and exercises only. An optician grinds lenses, fits them into frames, and adjusts the frames to the wearer.

CONTACT LENSES—HARD OR SOFT—SOMETIMES OR ALWAYS?

Many people are apprehensive about contact lenses—there is an almost primitive fear of putting anything in the eye. But they are really like a new window on the world for people with eye problems. There are two kinds of contact lenses. The hard contact lens has been used since about 1948, and it covers two-thirds of the cornea. It floats, like a piece of paper on water on a plate, on oxygen and new tears in front of the cornea.

The disadvantage of hard contact lenses is that you have to wear them regularly every day. If you stop wearing them, you have to build up to the wearing time again. In other words, you can't wear them one day for ten hours and the next day for two. It's like being in training—you have to wear them continuously. The wear and tear, however, is good—if you look after them well, they can last for years.

Soft contact lenses are a more recent development, and their advantage is that you can wear them one day for ten hours and the next day not at all. However, they do not give you the sharp vision that hard lenses give, and also the wear and tear is not so good. For instance, to take care of them you have to boil them every night for about twenty minutes. (New improved forms of sterilization are now being developed.) Also, if a patient has a certain amount of astigmatism, then he or she cannot wear soft contact lenses because the vision is not good enough—hard contact lenses would work better in this situation. (Astigmatism is where the curvature of one meridian of the eye is different from the curvature of the other meridian, so that you can focus on part of an object but not the whole.)

There are three main groups of people who may be prescribed contact lenses:

1. People who are myopic, that is, nearsighted.

2. People who have had cataract extraction or a corneal transplant.

3. People who have a deformity of the cornea or a scarring due to an accident or infection.

Farsighted individuals may also wear them, but this is not so common.

The prescription of the future

"Contact lenses are the prescription of the future," declares Dr. Jorge Buxton, surgeon, and Director of the Corneal Clinic at the New York Eye and Ear Infirmary. "The reasons are (a) cosmetic—so many people do not like to wear glasses, and (b) contact lenses, unlike glasses, do not reduce the visual field. People think of vision as looking straight ahead and seeing something with 20-20 accuracy, but actually much of our seeing is with our peripheral vision. A person can have an eye defect so that although he has 20-20 vision, he bumps into things.

"All it takes is motivation to wear them. Take a nearsighted girl: if she can recognize her boyfriend across the room at a cocktail party, even though he looks blurred, then she's not going to bother with contact lenses. If she has to put on her glasses to see him, then she's ready for contact lenses!"

The main reasons an ophthalmologist will not recommend contact lenses are: (a) lack of motivation; (b) the presence of certain diseases of the eye; and (c) if they are to be used only for reading.

Most people after forty have to wear reading glasses. What happens is that your zoom lens—the mechanism that helps you focus—becomes more static. The muscle works just as well as it always did, but the lens hardens. In this situation, glasses work fine, because you only need them at certain times—if you wore contact lenses for this purpose then you would not see well at a distance. (Bifocal contact lenses are, however, beginning to be prescribed.)

New developments in optical science

Dr. Buxton believes that the big thing in contact lenses of the future is going to be permanent wear—leaving them in for weeks and months. There are now experimental soft contact lenses that can work like this, and they are disposable.

The subject of contact lenses is a complicated one, and yet the more we know about it, the better for your eyes. In 1956 the National Eye Research Foundation was founded to do vision research and education for just this purpose. The National Director of the Foundation is optometrist Dr. Newton K. Wesley.

Dr. Wesley has a special interest in contact lenses He suffered from an eye defect called keratoconus, a condition in which the cornea becomes increasingly warped, and he pioneered a special kind of contact lens to correct this. "With advances in optical science," he says, "and with the help of a computer, which can calculate in seconds what a doctor would calculate in two years, we are now developing bifocal and multifocal lenses." Dr. Wesley himself wears a multifocal lens—a prescription that could only work in a contact lens. (It would not work in glasses because of the distance between them and your eye—multifocal eyeglasses would simply make you feel seasick, as your vision would wobble.)

Contact lenses are indeed the prescription of the future—one of the compensations of living in this advanced technological age.

THE SUNGLASSES SCENE

Most people own a pair of shades these days, whether for glamour, for anonymity, to intrigue people, to separate you from the world, to conceal wrinkles, or—their original purpose—to protect your eyes from glare.

What color suits you best?

"It used to be felt that certain colors, the pinks and the blues, for instance, were not only not helpful, but harmful," says Dr. William C. Cooper, Assistant Professor of Ophthalmology at Columbia Presbyterian Hospital, and in private practice in New York. "This is no longer felt to be true. The lighter tints filter less and are therefore less effective, but we no longer believe that they are harmful.

"Wearing tinted glasses depends upon the environment in which you wish to wear them. At the beach, on the water, or skiing, where the glare is particularly strong, a very dark tint is required. For normal city wearing, where there's a great deal of shadow and not a lot of direct or reflected light, then such a dark tint is not necessary.

"The amount of tint is registered by the percentage of filtration of light—*and for very bright light, as at the beach or on ski slopes, upwards of 85 percent filtration is required to get glare protection.* This is a very dark tint—so dark that you cannot see a person's eyes through the glasses, and so dark that you cannot wear them indoors without groping your way around.

"And this is where choice of color is important—the only two colors that will tint this dark are browns and grays. The other colors cannot be as densely tinted, so are unsuitable for very bright glare." (Gray also most accurately reproduces the actual color spectrum. American Optical's line of gray lenses is called "True Color.")

A changing tint?

The latest sunglasses discovery on the market is the photochromic lens—a glass that is impregnated with a photosensitive substance so that when light strikes the lens it darkens. These lenses come in two degrees—a lesser amount of photochromic substance in one makes it wearable indoors and outdoors when light is not too bright; then there's a stronger photochromic lens that can be used exclusively outdoors, going from a medium tint to a very dense tint. (These new lenses, however, cannot quite achieve the 85 percent filtration required in very bright glare, so they do not give perfect protection.)

One of the most dramatic improvements provided by these new photochromic lenses is in the field of indoor glare—particularly fluorescent. "Most people who complain of indoor lighting difficulties are suffering from fluorescent glare," says Dr. Cooper. "Photochromic lenses have been very helpful for this, and for indoor glare of any kind, because as the amount of glare intensifies, the degree of tint in the lens increases. Pale tinted glasses in any color can also help prevent this kind of glare—even the pinks, blues, and greens."

So those delicately hued glasses people are attracted to have some therapeutic as well as cosmetic use. But do be careful about what color you choose for your tint. What may look a wonderful match with your wardrobe may do very strange things to your mind. In an experiment on a mink farm in Cary, Illinois, it was found that the minks exposed to light through a deep pink glass became increasingly aggressive, difficult to manage, and in many instances actually vicious. Whereas when some of the minks were placed behind deep blue plastic they became friendly and docile. "The psychiatric literature is filled with reports that red is a vibrant, stimulating color," says Dr. Cooper. "Blue is more placid and soothing."

PLASTIC OR GLASS?

The Federal Government now requires *all* lenses be impact-resistant, but this means glass has to be specially treated, making it heavier. Perhaps you will be able to choose from looking at this chart:

GLASS		PLASTIC	
Advantages	**Disadvantages**	**Advantages**	**Disadvantages**
Cheaper Doesn't scratch	Heavier Less accurate prescription	Very light More accurate prescription	Scratches easily More expensive

HOW BIG IS BEAUTIFUL?

"The eye, when wearing spectacles, gets accustomed to the size lens that the eye is continually exposed to," explains Dr. Cooper. "And the size of these lenses is usually governed by the frame one chooses to wear. The lenses are made from a base curve to which the eye gets used. Now, if you dramatically change the base curve of the lens you wear, even if the prescription is not altered in any way, you may have a great deal of difficulty in adjusting to this new base curve." In other words, if you put on very large glasses after being accustomed to small ones, you may become nauseated, dizzy, and unhappy. If you stick with them, and don't change back, then the eye can adjust. But be consistent.

The size of your glasses depends, of course, on the frame

you choose. If possible, try on several types of frame in front of a full-length mirror—look for a shape that complements your facial structure. Try smiling with them on to see whether they hit your cheeks or ride up. Look down to the floor to see if they ride down your nose. If so, they need adjustment. If you are going to use them for sporting activities or driving, check to see that the peripheral side vision is good.

For those who wear contact lenses, the same rules about tint apply as for glasses. Dr. Cooper almost always prescribes tinted contact lenses for two reasons: "One, they are easier to see if they get lost, and two, because people who wear contact lenses are usually light-sensitive at first, since they are not accustomed to them—so a small degree of tint is helpful. A light tint can be worn indoors or out, the very dark tints can only be worn outdoors and must be changed as soon as you come inside."

One more tip—if you are nearsighted, you are likely to be more light-sensitive than a farsighted person, because generally speaking, nearsighted people's pupils are larger and therefore gather more light.

SPECIAL NOTE FOR BLUE EYES

Did you know that blue eyes were the most sensitive? Not only to *light*—because they contain less pigment than brown eyes and can't absorb so well—but also to *touch*. An ophthalmologist in a survey in Great Britain recently found that the corneas of people with blue eyes are more sensitive to touch than those of people with brown eyes (thus confirming what has been suspected by doctors fitting patients with contact lenses). So, combining all this together, what have we got? Blue-eyed, nearsighted people are the ones who *really* need good sunglasses to protect them from glare!

Chapter 9

SECRETS OF A RADIANT SMILE

A radiant smile may be the reflection of the inner you, but the wonderful white teeth that go with it are a reflection of nothing else except good, lifelong tooth care. It's the part we see that we care most about—the hopefully white part, made of enamel, the hardest substance of the body. Most people now know that tooth care does not just mean clean white teeth, it also means healthy gums.

TOOTH-TELLING

"If one supports the theory that teeth grew in an evolutionary fashion in response to need, then it would follow that our teeth would now be growing less important, as our diet changes," says Dr. Irwin D. Mandel, Professor of Dentistry and Director of the Division of Preventive Dentistry, Columbia University School of Dental and Oral Surgery. "But the closest one may come to this is the observation that there seem to. be more people born with missing wisdom teeth today. The latest figures suggest that up to 17 percent of the population may have missing wisdom teeth. This may be because we don't need them—we do our chewing with our first and second molars.

"In fact wisdom teeth are perhaps nature's gift of a third set of teeth, the first set being our baby teeth, the second set growing at about age six, so that at age twelve we have twenty-eight adult teeth, with four more to fill in the back spaces even later—the wisdom teeth. The reason why we have two sets is because of the growth of the human head— had we been born with a full complement of adult teeth, there would be no room for anything else! Lower forms, such as sharks, grow constant sets of successive teeth."

THE DANGERS

There are two basic threats to shining white teeth—dental decay and pyorrhea (gum disease, also known as gingivitis). Dental decay deals with the destruction of the teeth, pyorrhea with the destruction of the gums. Yet they have one thing in common. Both come about as the result of the action of clumps of bacteria known as plaque. "In the case of dental decay, the plaque that we are interested in is on the inside surface of these clumps of bacteria facing the tooth," explains Dr. Mandel. "In gum disease we are concerned with the outer surface, where a variety of toxic substances are formed, which can cause inflammation and break down gum tissue. This plaque also becomes hardened and calcifies to form tartar, or calculus, also accelerating gum disease."

The average seventeen-year-old American has 8.7 filled, decayed, or missing teeth, according to the National Institute of Dental Research. Tooth decay afflicts at least 95 percent of Americans, most of them children and young adults. If you are past thirty-five, the teeth you lose will most likely be lost to gum disease. In short, it's time to join the fight against plaque—and if you do succeed, even partially, then there is a great chance that you can save your teeth from further damage and can flash that radiant smile well into old age.

HOW TO BEAT PLAQUE

1. Identify plaque. Do this by staining your teeth with one of the disclosing tablets now in drugstores (you can get red or green ones). This is important, because unless you know where it is, you cannot try to remove it by brushing. Chew the tablet or rinse your mouth with it, and you will see stains left on your teeth—this is where the plaque is. Now, when you brush your teeth, you can check to see if you are removing the stain. If there are no stains, you have succeeded!

2. Brush properly. The major weapon in plaque removal is still the toothbrush. The revolution, however, has been that the brush is now seen primarily not as a method to make teeth look white, but as an efficient plaque remover. Much plaque concentrates round the gum line at an angle. There are now multitufted, soft nylon bristle brushes with rounded tips, so that when you angle the brush to remove the plaque from along the gum line, you are not damaging the gum tissue. These are the best buy. Choose a handle that you can move around your mouth comfortably—if you have a small mouth, you must use a smaller brush and handle. Even a children's brush is often recommended.

3. Use fluoride. The various applications of fluoride can really protect the teeth and gums from much potential damage. Fluoride in drinking water, for instance, can become part of the blood stream and find its way into the bones and teeth, with a resulting 60 percent reduction in tooth decay. Fluoride has been the savior when it comes to teeth, counteracting the damage done by sugar and the accumulation of plaque. Fluoride toothpaste can produce a 20 percent reduction in decay. In addition, dentists can prescribe mouthwashes and a new fluoride gel in a plastic tray that is placed against the tooth. This new process can be done at home once a day or week with excellent results,

especially with children or adults with a high incidence of tooth decay.

The plastic tray is probably the most effective anti-decay procedure we have today—the results suggest about 85 percent reduction. You build so much fluoride into the tooth's surface that you build its resistance, something of particular value in an area where the water is not fluoridated. (Less than half the population enjoys fluoride in drinking water. A lot of cities still turn it down, although for thirty years it has been found effective and endorsed by the American Dental Association. The controversy still rages.)

Pure fluoride, however, cannot be purchased over the counter, though the FDA is reevaluating it. For now, your dentist must prescribe any of the applications using fluoride— except of course, fluoride in toothpaste—such as mouthwashes, tablets, chewable lozenges, and the plastic tray.

4. Watch your diet. An adequate diet is essential in order to provide the optimum resistance of the teeth and gums to disease. Some practitioners claim that a higher dose of calcium, phosphorus, vitamins C, A, and D, is more advantageous for tooth and gum health. This is very controversial, and for every study that claims this, ten prove that it makes no difference. Research in this field is currently being carried out all over the country. At the moment, Dr. Mandel would advise that people not experiment with megavitamins until more evidence can be collected.

The thing that everyone is agreed upon, however, is that too much sugar and carbohydrates are definitely bad, and that reducing the intake of sugar will reduce the amount of plaque and acid in the mouth.

5. Use floss. The value of floss is that it reaches where the toothbrush can't reach—between the teeth especially near the gum line.

Break off about 18 inches of floss and wind the ends round your middle fingers. Use your thumbs and forefingers with an inch of floss between them to guide the floss between your teeth. Hold the floss tightly and use a gentle sawing motion to insert it between the teeth, then work it up and down against the side of the tooth. Repeat this on all your teeth. Floss should never be snapped or forced between teeth and into gum margins.

OTHER AIDS

Plastic sealants. The idea is that coating the surface of the tooth with plastic will protect the enamel against decay. The only coatings used now are placed on the biting surfaces of the back teeth, and are indeed of some benefit in preventing plaque, as these areas are hard to reach with brushes, and especially in young people, these teeth are prone to decay. However, we have only been using them for up to three years—so we have no information yet on long-term use. Over 80 percent of sealants will last three years and reduce decay; that is as much as we know.

Electric toothbrushes. This makes little difference, because if you brush in a hurry, you brush in just as much of a hurry with the electric brush. Where it can be of benefit is for people who have difficulties holding a small brush or making hand movements, such as arthritics.

Mouth hygiene equipment. This equipment washes out toxic materials; so it can rinse out effectively places that are hard to reach with the brush, especially if you have gum disease.

Chewing gum. Regular chewing gum has approximately a teaspoon of sugar in it, so that is bad. But there is also an increase in salivary stimulation because of the chewing, which cleans out the mouth—so if you only use it occasionally the cleansing can balance out the sugar. It is when it's used as candy that it can be harmful. Sugar-free gums are of course far preferable.

HOW TO BRUSH YOUR TEETH

1. Apply the toothbrush to the outside tooth surfaces at about a 45-degree angle directed toward the area where teeth and gums meet. Press so as to slide the bristles against the teeth at the gum line. (The tufts of the bristles should divide to "straddle" the gum line.)

2. In this position, move the brush back and forth with *short* (half-a-tooth-wide) strokes several times, using a gentle "scrubbing" motion. Brush the outer surfaces of all your teeth in this method, keeping the bristles angled against the gum line. Use the same method for the inside of the teeth.

3. For the front teeth, brush the inside surfaces of the upper and lower jaws by tilting the brush vertically and making several gentle up-and-down strokes with the front part of the brush as well as side-to-side motions.

(These instructions are currently recommended by the American Dental Association to remove plaque.)

Chapter 10

HANDS UP FOR HEALTH

SURGEON'S Rx FOR HANDS

Dr. Richard G. Eaton of the world-famous Hand Service, Department of Surgery at Roosevelt Hospital in New York City, talks about the structure of the hand and gives first-aid tips.

"The hand is our connection with our environment. We may look at and hear things, but there's no contact involved in the literal sense of the word. When it comes to manipulating and doing things, the hand and the sense of touch are the final common pathways. The hands are miniaturized machines capable of an almost infinite number of combinations of positions that apply power with precision:

—Each hand contains 27 bones in all: 8 wrist bones, 5 in the palm, and 14 in all five fingers. Two hands equal 54 bones, which is a quarter of all the bones in the skeleton.
—The hand contains the most densely packed system of nerve endings in the body.
—The thumb alone does 45 percent of the hand's work.
—A strong man can develop his grip to equal 120 pounds; a strong woman can build her grip to about half this.
—The two largest areas of the cerebral cortex are reserved for right- and left-hand motor action.
—Nature has equipped the hand by giving it two of almost everything it uses to insure its functioning—two nerves in

each finger, as well as two tendons and two veins. If any one of these is cut, function, though inhibited, is still maintained. —Modern surgical techniques can fashion a thumb from an index finger. The tendons in the hand are flexible and can be shifted to permit this kind of borrowing.

"Electric tools present the most common danger to the hand. By concentrating on what you're doing when you use them you're less likely to have accidents of this type.

"A blister should be left intact. The 'shell' over the blister is usually sufficient covering to protect the hand from infection. If the blister ruptures, simply wash with water and apply a soothing dressing so that the new skin can grow.

"Try to remove splinters if you can. The old saying that a splinter will be absorbed into the bloodstream is incorrect. Splinters don't migrate. It may be carried out of the hand on a drop of serum if the splinter is accompanied by infection. Otherwise it stays put and will probably become infected. Soften the skin around it with water and remove it with tweezers. If the splinter is 'buried,' take it to a doctor as some splinters can contribute to blood poisoning.

"When a puncture occurs try to make it bleed and wash with water. If you can't, try to get to a doctor for a tetanus booster.

"Should you drop a heavy object on a fingertip, first apply ice for about four to eight hours to reduce any internal bleeding. Then apply heat to dilate the blood vessels and carry off stagnated blood tissues and promote the free flow of blood. A painful swelling of a joint may indicate a sprained finger. Again cold water or ice will reduce the swelling. Until you can get to a doctor, tie the finger to an adjacent finger to help keep it straight."

HANDCARE SECRETS FROM CRAFTSMEN

Mary Cara, basketweaver: "I sometimes get tiny bramble prickers in my fingertips. A needle or tweezers usually gets them out. Otherwise I just rub A&D Ointment on before and after I work. Something about the weaving itself seems to be keeping my hands soft and smooth. Maybe the rough reeds and grasses help to remove that dead surface layer of skin."

Eleanor Weller, furniture refinisher: "I always keep a garden hose running whenever I'm working with abrasive chemicals outdoors. That way an accidental spill can be immediately rinsed off. There are about six thicknesses of rubber gloves that I use also, each a size larger than my hand. It's for the same reason. If a chemical were to leak through, the glove can be whisked off instantly."

Hannah Wister, gardener: "I just dig my nails into a dry cake of soap before I go out to work in the soil. The dirt couldn't be easier to wash away after."

Gigs Stevens, bargello embroiderer: "A tailor's open-ended thimble goes over my middle finger and helps prevent calluses from the needle. And when working with a brand new canvas it helps to roll it back and forth a few times to help get the 'starch' out. The canvas won't warp and it will be somewhat softer on your hands."

Richard Neas, crewel embroiderer: "My index finger which holds the embroidery material underneath my needle some-times feels like a sieve from all the pricking it gets. I need that finger bare to use as a guide for the placement of the needle and to push it back up through the fabric. My solution is simply use hand cream that sinks into the skin and helps soothe that part of my finger."

Sol Kent, needlepoint embroiderer: "I leave my hands com-pletely to nature. There's a thick callus on my finger and I just let it alone. No creams or special lotions. I don't mind."

A DERMATOLOGIST'S OUNCE OF PREVENTION

Norman Orentreich, M.D., Clinical Associate Professor of

Dermatology at New York University Medical School, discusses proper nail and skin care:

"Manicuring has to be done carefully. Excessive paring of the tissues around the cuticle can allow infections to start and pressure against the skin at the base of the nail can affect the 'matrix,' or growing portion.

"The hand's nails grow about a millimeter a week. Nails involved in activity, such as typing, grow faster than nails that aren't. They'll grow faster on the side on which you are 'handed', in warmer climates, and during pregnancy. You can expect, on the average, though, about three months for a completely new set of nails.

"Some of the things you can do to protect your nails are simple: Use a pushbutton telephone or do your dialing with a pencil; don't insert the nail into anything; use the pads of your fingers to pick things up; use protective scouring pads for pots and pans; and wear gloves when you're doing really coarse work; and find the best length for your nails—consider what they have to do as well as how they look.

"Hand creams are invaluable for good hand care. And when you work outdoors get hand creams that contain sunscreens. If you've been recently exposed to a great deal of sunlight and you find that a blemish on the back of the hand is becoming annoying, take it to a dermatologist.

"Pass up gloves unless you're working with chemicals or sharp objects. I feel that gloves diminish the sensitivity of the hands and fingers and the perspiration that accumulates in the linings of gloves provides needless irritations that can be difficult to contend with."

THE FINISHING TOUCH—MANICURE TIPS

From Saks Fifth Avenue's manicurist Corinne Caduff:

1. Use nail polish removers that contain added "oils."

2. Cover the tip of your orange stick with a bit of cotton.

3. If you push your cuticle back with a finger instead of an

orange stick, cover the index finger with the tip of a terry towel.

4. Use a base coat when you apply polish. It's designed to protect the nails from chemicals in the polish.

5. Wait 6 or 7 hours before wetting freshly polished nails.

6. Snip away dead skin or hangnails. Avoid cutting the cuticle.

METS' DOCTOR ON THE BASEBALL HAND

Dr. James C. Parkes II, Orthopedic Surgeon for the New York Mets, tells how his players' hands can help you keep yours at their best.

"Baseball is a game of fine timing, split-second timing, in fact, and it can't be played well unless the hands are in excellent health. The tiniest, most insignificant cut that you and I wouldn't bother much about is a matter of crucial concern to a baseball player and especially a pitcher.

"Ordinary friction causes calluses. When the callus goes too deep, layers of skin may begin to move over on top of each other with a painful fluid build-up in between. We file calluses dry with a sandpaper file that looks very much like a woman's emery board only bigger. Otherwise rest is the best remedy—but try to recommend rest to active people.

"We keep the players' nails short to avoid breaking and tearing. Other than that, they're pretty much on their own.

"Some players feel that their hands and wrist are stronger when they wear a wrist-strap. As long as there is no fracture a wrist-strap is fine. The benefit may be more of a psychological crutch than some players care to admit, but if a stable, rigid wrist makes a sportsman or athlete more comfortable, then let him or her wear a strap."

Dr. Parkes suggests that everyone keep the following in a *first-aid kit for hands:* shaped, sterile dressings that fit over the fingers and into the palms; betadine ointment or solution for blisters, small cuts, scrapes, abrasions; manicuring scissors; surgical tape; tongue depressors to make a temporary splint for a bruised finger; and emery boards for broken nails and thickening calluses.

HERE'S THE RUB—STEP-BY-STEP HAND MASSAGE

Vicki Schick of the Profile Health Spa in New York City shows you how to give one to yourself. How often should you have it? Whenever you feel like it or whenever hands have been doing an activity for a while.

1. Slather fingers, hand, and wrist with hand lotion. Use a lotion that's fairly thin. Rosewater and glycerin has both the emollients needed for lubrication and water to help keep skin slick during the massage.

2. Starting with the outside knuckles of the little finger or the index finger, gently but firmly massage the area in between the knuckles. Work each side toward the center with palm down.

3. From the center knuckle space gently massage the bones of the hand to the wrist. You should feel the surface of each fingerbone and the tension between the bones begin to ease as you get closer to the wrist.

4. Turn the palm up and massage the pulse area.

5. At the web of the little finger begin to stroke finger toward fingertip; repeat for each finger and thumb. Give a gentle squeeze at the tips. Stroking the fingers should also include a slight pulling. Rotate fingers and thumb twice in each direction and finish with a gentle tug.

6. Open palm and roll fingers of opposite hand and briskly rub the open palm.

7. Dab massaging fingers with a bit more lotion and massage into the cuticle area of each nail.

8. Grasp the wrist and with the whole hand gently pull down the length of the hand. Fingers should be gently squeezed together. Repeat for opposite hand.

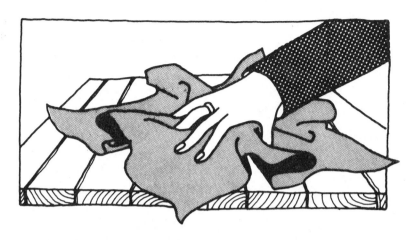

DEXTERITY IMPROVER

Lay a flat sheet of newspaper on a table and with one hand only reach, stretch, grasp, and crumple it into a ball. The weightless paper allows for full flexing and stretching of the fingers and wrist muscles.
Dr. James Parkes, Orthopedic Surgeon for the New York Mets

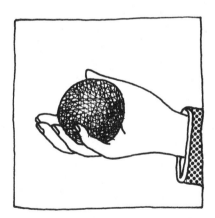
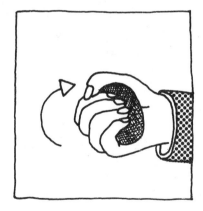

STRENGTH BUILDERS

A 2½-inch rubber ball will help develop your grip. Squeeze and release over and over again until the wrist and fingers feel slightly tired. Stop. Once in the morning and again at night will strengthen muscles in the wrist and those extending from the top and bottom of the elbow.
Marjorie Craig

Chapter 11

THE CROWNING GLORY

Shiny, bouncy hair is a pleasure to look at and a sign of inner health. In fact, you can't have one without the other. That's why it is to the most distinguished medical specialists that the wise crowning-glory hunter turns, rather than a shampoo artist. What happens in the beauty parlor is merely the icing on top of the cake.

THE SCIENCE OF HAIR

Ronald L. Rizer is a biochemist. He works with the world-famous Orentreich Medical Group in New York City, specializing in hair disorders. Mr. Rizer works behind the scenes, in a laboratory, doing major research in the molecular biology of hair growth. That's the kind of expert your hair needs.

"Your hair," he begins, "is dead. Completely dead. But the follicle in the skin that produces this by-product, hair, is very much alive. In fact, it's one of the most active tissues in the body. All of the dead material that we call hair is really protein that has been synthesized by the live hair follicle.

"Every hair in the scalp goes through a cycle. There's a growing phase, called anagen, and a resting phase, called telogen. The growing phase for scalp hairs in humans varies roughly from 2 to 5 years. They grow about 6 inches every year. This phase is followed by the resting phase of some 3 to

6 months, when the hair does not increase in length and the attachment of the hair to the base of the follicle becomes progressively weaker. Finally, as a result of ordinary wear and tear, its own weight, and the push from a new hair growing up, the old hair is shed. The average human scalp has approximately 100,000 hairs.

"The human hair cycle is random, rather than seasonal. About 90 percent of the follicles are in the growing phase at one time while the other 10 percent are resting. This produces an average daily replacement of 100 hairs."

Mr. Rizer adds this comment: "There's a vast difference between talking about dead hair and talking about living hair follicles."

Now this may seem an innocuous enough remark. But in fact it is the key to the other part of this true story about your hair.

THE AMAZING SCALP

Dr. Norman Orentreich, Director of the Orentreich Medical Group and Associate Clinical Professor of Dermatology, New York University School of Medicine, treats diseases of the scalp. The scalp is skin and very sensitive. "The scalp, for instance," says Dr. Orentreich, "is one of the most prevalent places for psoriasis and dermatitis. Most people are not aware of this; if they had the same amount of dermatitis on their face, they'd run to a doctor. If it's on their scalp, they run to a hair salon. Probably most beauty salons will recognize a medical scalp problem when they see it, which needs medical treatment. But that's not most people's problem; they just don't know how to take care of their hair properly."

In other words, treating the scalp is one thing, treating the hair is another. The scalp is live tissue; the hair is dead.

"Once it leaves your scalp it's as inert as a wool sweater," explains Dr. Orentreich. "Now if you wore that wool sweater every day, you wore it in the sun, you bathed in it, for three years, what do you think it would look like by now? It would be pretty frayed. You can do anything you like to that sweater, but you cannot recondition it. The same thing with hair. Once you have fraying, and split ends, the best thing is to cut it back, to a healthier level, to the newer hair."

Hair is unbelievably durable, Dr. Orentreich points out. Mummies have been dug up after 2,000 years and they still have hair. But we do cruel things to it. We leave it in the sun. We put chemicals on it, which break up the protein. We wave, bleach, straighten, dye, curl. Every one of these manipulations weakens the body of the hair. Think of giving that treatment to your three-year-old sweater.

The conclusion of all this presents the romantically un-clouded truth. The best and happiest hair in the world would be kept clean and well conditioned, and remain otherwise untouched by human hand or chemical alteration—then it would grow as long and glossy as you wanted.

But who is going to settle for what she's got? Hardly anyone. It's no *fun* anyway. Meanwhile, perhaps knowing some of the myths about hair will allow the best possible version of your crowning glory to be shown to the world.

FOUR MYTHS ABOUT HAIR

Myth 1: Shampooing is bad for the hair. Wrong. "Hair was designed to protect mammals from water and exposure," says Dr. Orentreich. "It takes cleansing well. One should sham-poo regularly. The best shampoos are mild, the ones that babies can use. Unless you need a medicated shampoo for a problem scalp. If you worry about hair in the tub—that's normal. Those 100 hairs a day, plus some of tomorrow's, are being shed."

Myth 2: Brushing 100 times a day is good. Wrong. "Even with the best of brushes, one should not brush or comb except to groom: 100 strokes a day simply pulls out hair."

Myth 3: Vigorous scalp massage is good. Wrong. "There is no way of increasing the blood supply sufficiently to the scalp by massage. Vigorous massage will rip out more hair than it will grow."

Myth 4: "Feeding" the hair with protein or egg is good. Wrong. "The hair is dead. You can't feed it from outside. Such treatments merely wash out with the next shampoo. The best conditioners are the standard ones, which contain pH neutralization (acid), sheen, antistatic action, better slip. You can't restructure your wool sweater or your hair. Simply minimize the damage by standard conditioning and shampooing."

Dr. Orentreich again remarks how wonderfully durable the human hair is. "I'm not against the things people do to their hair," he declares. "Naturally you want to look your best and feel your best. But don't change your mind every week. Allow your hair judicious coloring, judicious waving, judicious bleaching, judicious straightening—the word 'judicious' is everything."

HIS & HER HAIR—WHY SOME GROWS & SOME GOES

Why men go bald and women, on the whole, do not, is one of those imponderables that still elude the investigations of scientists, biologists, and doctors. Men's hair roots, that is the follicles in a male scalp, are no different, it seems, from women's. If you put a hair under a microscope, no expert could tell whether it came from a man or a woman. The only thing doctors can say is that there is a male and female pattern of hair growth; men are potentially subject to male-pattern baldness, and women, with some exceptions, are not.

Why do men go bald? Dr. Robert A. Berger, a dermatologist interested in both male and female hair disorders, and Assistant Professor at Mount Sinai College of Medicine in New York City, says, "It is simply a sex characteristic, peculiar only in that it affects just a minority of men. If all men went bald at about the same age, just as they grow a beard, then nobody would worry. It would be accepted as a male characteristic. But because it only hits a certain number, and because most men lose more hair as they get older, baldness is regarded as abnormal; and it also becomes psychologically associated with aging, therefore is thought by many to be socially undesirable."

Before women start crowing, however, let it be said that many women also suffer from hair loss—but luckily, they tend to lose it in a less noticeable way. "Women don't usually show a bald spot on the top of their heads or a recession at the peaks of their foreheads, as men do," explains Dr. Berger, "but rather they show a thinning all over the scalp. For this reason you don't commonly see as much baldness in women as you do men. But millions of young and middle-aged women show a degree of hair loss that is at least enough to be disturbing to them. It's very common."

This form of hair loss in women seems to be the same as in men—inexplicable and unstoppable. What happens is that the hair follicles in the scalp gradually start shrinking, so that each generation of hair that grows is a little finer than the one before and grows for a shorter time. Ultimately the hairs become so small that they can only be seen through a magnifying glass. The effect is baldness. The hair follicles have not died; they are still there—only for some reason the shed hair does not grow again. Nobody has been successful yet in growing hair again from these follicles.

The woman's angle

There are many other reasons why women shed hair—apart from the obvious damage caused by too much bleaching or perming. The following types of hair loss are *temporary,* caused by some specific change in a person's metabolism. The hair will usually find its normal cycle of good growing and resting phases after a few months. There are three common causes:

1. Trauma. Any severe shock to the system by illness or trauma can put the hair into the resting stage (telogen); thus the normal cycle is disrupted and hair falls out. For instance, a girl who goes on a crash diet and eats only vitamins for a month may well find that a month later her hair starts falling out, because of the metabolic shock to her system. But it's only temporary—the hair soon grows back.

2. Pregnancy. At this time, hair follicles stay longer in the growing phase, with less shedding than usual. After the birth, they move into telogen, thus causing more shedding after about three months, all at the same time. After a while the cycle then returns to its normal "staggered" timing.

3. Going off the contraceptive pill. Taking the pill is being, in a sense, in a state of permanent pregnancy. If you stop taking the pill, after a couple of months you may notice hair loss, just as after pregnancy. But this, too, is temporary. The hair soon grows back.

Sex and the single hair

Pregnancy, pills, hormonal changes ... What effect *do* hormones have on hair growth?

If you took a panel of normal women and deliberately gave them large amounts of male hormone, they would almost all grow beards. This means that hair growth on the face is a male characteristic that requires male hormone. Women have the same potential to grow facial hair, but normally they do not have the necessary amount of male hormone to bring it out (unless they have some gland disorder or tumor, which temporarily increases male hormone).

As well as growing beards, about one-third of them will start to show a male-pattern baldness. This means that the normal women we have described as suffering from a gradual form of permanent baldness probably started out with a susceptibility to hair loss, and that the normal amount of male hormone for a woman (about two-thirds of a man's) is enough to cause some degree of hair loss for these women.

According to Dr. Berger, in this situation, adjustment of hormones *can* make a difference. "The conclusion I favor," he says, "after many years' study along with Dr. Norman Orentreich and others, is that estrogen (female hormone) can help women suffering from a slow, progressive hair loss over many years." It is also possible that female hormone could help male baldness, but the amount required to be effective would also feminize them in other respects (enlarging breasts) so this treatment cannot be considered practical. "Not every woman should take estrogen," Dr. Berger adds, "but it can be helpful and safe."

Chapter 12

YOU AND YOUR DOCTOR

Knowing something about how your body works is one thing. Knowing how your doctor works is another. People so often feel that the doctor knows secrets he isn't telling—that the consulting room is a frightening place—that science is moving too fast in medicine. Here are three basic questions you probably always wanted to ask your doctor but never got round to it, answered by Dr. Mary Catherine Tyson.

Q. What would a doctor list as the main dos and don'ts for healthy living?
A. As you read each of these nine essentials ask yourself: "Have I given this enough thought?"

1. Steer clear of all medicines, and all drugs, unless prescribed. (Obvious exceptions are mild pain relievers and digestive remedies.) Even aspirin, taken continuously and in large quantities, can cause stomach hemorrhages.

2. A reasonable balance of four vital nutritional elements: proteins, vitamins, minerals, roughage. No extreme diets, regardless of who recommends them, without your doctor's OK.

3. Alcoholic drinks in moderation. Too much alcohol can contribute to dietary deficiencies and cause other damage to the system.

4. Do you now weigh about what you should have weighed at age twenty? If not, zero in on that number starting today,

on your own or with your doctor's plan. Overweight causes and aggravates so many troubles there's no space to list them. Reduced life expectancy is´one dramatic effect. Better appearance and more comfort are enough reward by themselves. Remember, it is physical appearance which first attracts men and women to each other because it has a stimulating hint of sex adventure. No crash diet or superhuman effort! A pound a week will do it more reliably.

5. Better muscle tone, heart function, good (and good-looking!) posture will be your prizes if you take suitable exercise. Excess body fat and flabbiness will be minimized. Your age and life situation determine the best exercise for you. Competitive sports like golf and tennis have the best interest value. However, you can jog and perform otherwise indoors without special clothing and in all sorts of weather. Radio news and music reduce boredom. Timing and other ways of measuring your progress can help to motivate you. Your doctor can prescribe exercise if you inquire.

6. Rest isn't just a pleasure, it's a must. Seven or eight hours of sleep should do it. You don't need more and those extra hours slow your circulation.

7. Think twice before you pick up the next cigarette. The Surgeon General has determined that cigarette smoking endangers your health.

8. Let your doctor and dentist see you each year. Don't put it off because you worry about what they might find or because you have symptoms that seem scary. The anxiety of not knowing—not to speak of not getting treatment if needed—is much worse than getting it settled.

9. Enjoy your good health. Asked "What's the most important thing in your life?" most people say "My health!" That's what they say, but just about every one of them takes good health for granted and doesn't really appreciate it. Seeing,

hearing, smelling, tasting, being able to stand, walk, bend over, and sit comfortably—these are all wonderful abilities! The whole sensation of well-being, not hurting, is one of life's treasures. To recapture this feeling, think back to when you were last ill, how you longed simply to be well. Every morning, think about that feeling.

Q. How can I be sure my doctor is giving me a thorough physical checkup?
A. No one should assume that a doctor has done a complete physical examination. Sometimes vital points may be neglected. All sixteen items listed below, depending on your age, are significant parts of the exam. When you have your yearly checkup discuss them. If the doctor is the right person for you, you'll probably get a pleasant answer, though you shouldn't be put off by a mild show of indignation.

Your complete physical includes: Urine analysis. Blood pressure readings. Measurement of weight. Hemoglobin test for possible anemia. Careful examination of nose, throat, eyes. Palpation, or feeling, of neck for glands or thyroid nodules. Examination of lungs and heart with stethoscope. Careful palpation of abdomen to check for enlargement of organs, masses, hernia. Checking of reflexes with rubber hammer. Examination of skin (with patient in medical gown only), so entire skin surface can be checked for growth and general condition.

For female patients: Examination of breasts with patient sitting up and lying down. "Pap" test for cancer detection, based on smear of the pelvic organs.

For patients over fifty: Stool test for detection of cancer of the intestinal tract. Rectal examination, including (for males) prostate exam. Blood sugar and cholesterol test. Electrocardiogram (earlier than fifty, if heart symptoms are present).

From this general checkup, further tests (such as X rays) can be made if indicated.

Q. Is scientific analysis by computer going to replace conventional diagnosis in the doctor's office?

A. Computerized diagnosis, radioactive isotopes, and scanning are among the marvels of today's medical profession, but the most refined diagnostic instrument remains the doctor's ear. Given a choice of physical examination, a complex laboratory workup, or a personal history, most internists agree that the personally taken history is the best single method of producing accurate diagnosis. An expensive, elaborate lab workup may actually miss a significant clue to understanding an illness. Example: A woman with convulsions was hospitalized as an emergency at midnight. Neither an angiogram nor the range of neurological X rays revealed the cause. Her family physician, contacted later, listened. After talking to the patient and hearing that she had had a strenuous day at work, skipped lunch, eaten a skimpy dinner to get to the theater on time, then rushed home to avoid a snowstorm, the doctor ordered a simple sugar tolerance test. The result showed a case of hypoglycemia (low blood sugar), easily treated by diet. A week in the hospital might easily have been avoided.

It is in the patient's best interest to have a doctor who both listens and explains. For the listening doctor, one patient's migraine is a treatable allergy, while another's is an emotional reaction to persistent marital disagreement. If a question of surgery arises, it is important that the doctor explain the exact need for it in as much detail as possible. Lack of explanation leaves an uninformed patient more likely to be dissatisfied and sue for malpractice. (The rare haughty, aloof doctor can create such situations.) Personal communication in medicine is vital. A patient must understand his or her physical condition to take care of it and do well. The diabetic, for instance, should know almost as much about diabetes as the doctor does, something that can come about only through patient explanation in the doctor's office. Scientific aids are fine, but not as a substitute for sympathetic one-to-one contact. If you find it difficult to get attentive listening and suitable explanations from your doctor, it would be wise to find another.

Part Two

NUTRITION AND FUEL FOR A HEALTHY BODY

Today, good nutrition is recognized as one of the most important aspects of a healthy life. In these pages, you can learn how to eat right, what certain nutrients do for your body and where to find them, and what to feed your family, particularly young athletes, for maximum performance.

Chapter 13

HOW TO EAT, AND WHEN

by Eloise R. Trescher, R.D.

Oscar Wilde once described someone as knowing the price of everything and the value of nothing. This could refer to a lot of people nowadays when they talk about food. The rising cost of food is a Number 1 conversation piece, but so many don't realize that the right foods in the right amounts do help their bodies, and the lack of certain foods hinders healthy growth.

Fortunately for all of us, more and more articles and books are being written about nutrition, the study of *how* foods, once you've eaten them, help make you a healthy individual.

You can consume three wonderfully balanced meals each day, and be very proud of yourself, but you are still wasting your time if you gulp them in ten minutes flat. A meal should be treated as a graceful pause, not as if you were trying to break a track record.

For a change of pace, why not a different setting for your meals? The Roman general Lucullus had several dining rooms in his house so that meals of different degrees of luxury could be served with backgrounds appropriate to the person he was entertaining. That's exaggerating it a bit, I agree, but why not breakfast in bed *after* the children go to school? Why not a living room picnic dinner in the middle of the week?

Wherever you eat, you should give 60 to 90 minutes a day to eating. While spending more time eating, you extend the *pleasure* of it. You'll improve your digestion as well as help to reduce gas and burping, and prevent heartburn. You'll reduce calorie intake, improve the health of your gums and teeth, conserve food, save money, and if that's not enough, you might find yourself cultivating the art of cozy and informative communication with your family and guests. And eating slowly is a marvelous way to relax!

If you are a rapid eater, all of these benefits could be accomplished by allowing a minimum of twenty to thirty minutes for each meal, and by acquiring the practice of eating slowly, chewing each bite so thoroughly that the food will be finely divided when it reaches the second station in the stomach.

Comparatively few people take this advice seriously. Yet it is free for the taking. What is required is a retraining of your eating habits. A habit is established more easily if you believe it is a habit of value to yourself. It is repeated again and again until it becomes a fixed habit or way of life. By chewing food thoroughly you also may prevent that uncomfortable feeling of fullness after a meal. Other causes of indigestion in the healthy individual are emotional in origin such as built-up tensions and pressures. So why hurry? Give mealtimes priority. Relax and enjoy.

Thorough mastication exercises the gums and improves the blood supply to the teeth. It excites the secretion of saliva. Digestion begins in the mouth, and, if you don't chew slowly and well, the process of digestion will take longer. The stomach will have to work harder, contracting and expanding more to prepare the food for its further travel along the digestive tract. An enzyme in the saliva acts upon starch in the mouth and begins its conversion into maltose and dextrose.

Saliva prepares food for swallowing by changing its consistency and acting as a solvent. The more liquid the food, the more taste one experiences. Remember that chewing starts salivary secretion. The moistened food stimulates the taste buds, whch are on the tongue, and enhances the enjoyment of taste.

Saliva acts also as a cleansing agent. Particles of food allowed to stay in the mouth serve as an excellent "culture media" for the growth of bacteria. Saliva clears them away. Saliva moistens and lubricates the lips and mouth. This improves articulation and personal comfort. Saliva serves, too, as an excretory agent of many organic and inorganic substances, and plays a vital role in the regulation of water balance in the body.

Salivary secretion is activated as well by nerves and hormones. (The word "hormone" is derived from the Greek word meaning "to excite.") Materials placed in the mouth call forth after a short, latent period (two or three seconds) a secretion of saliva; which varies in quantity and quality with the physical and chemical nature of the substance introduced. And taste affects the secretion of saliva. Pleasant tastes are perhaps one of the most powerful salivary stimulants. Unpleasant tastes (inedible substances, strong acids) can and do cause profuse salivation.

Just as the real epicure swirls gently a superb vintage wine to savor the bouquet, then sips it slowly to enjoy the flavor to the fullest, so the real gourmet prolongs the pleasure of food by eating slowly. The gourmet never gobbles his food; only the gourmand does this. Large mouthfuls of food distort the face. More serious, a large bite of food swallowed without being finely divided by chewing and moistened by saliva may become lodged in the throat or esophagus and result in death.

People with gastritis, gastric or duodenal ulcers, hiatus hernia, diverticulosis, to mention a few, often find their discomfort is lessened and sometimes disappears entirely when they practice the simple act of eating slowly and chewing food thoroughly. Even if you don't have any of these ailments, you'll find the more slowly you eat, the less food you are likely to eat in a given time. Eating slowly is a great ruse for cutting down on total calorie intake without feeling deprived. By eating smaller quantities of food, we can reduce our food bills as well as effect a gradual reduction in weight.

Millions are spent each year on the care of the teeth. It is a sound investment. Much of the investment is initiated for comfort or cosmetic purposes. More importantly, teeth which do not occlude, or meet correctly, hamper proper chewing of foods. Remember the act of chewing "exercises" the teeth and improves the blood supply to the gums in which teeth are anchored.

"We dig our graves with our teeth" is an ancient and familiar adage. The implication is that we overeat, and many do. An additional hazard is that in failing to chew well we make a fertile bed for the development of many disorders, mainly digestive, which might with thorough mastication and relaxation be avoided. The moral is to eat slowly and foster this practice until it becomes a firmly established habit.

For the rapid eater, tricks to slow down the process often help. One is to lay down the knife, fork, or spoon between each bite and engage in conversation before the next bite. This practice is effective for many overweight individuals who stow away excessive quantities of food in an amazingly brief time. A second one is gradually to decrease the quantities of food provided, and a third, of course, is no second helpings.

A patient of mine lost weight by having the platter of meat placed at the opposite end of the table in front of his wife where he could not contemplate, cut off, and eat the choice morsels that he enjoyed. When he stopped eating those small, high-calorie snacks throughout the meal, he discovered that he not only felt better but his heartburn and feeling of fullness disappeared too. And his girth gradually diminished. Such benefits are not accomplished in a day, a week, nor a month. Substituting and implementing a good habit for a poor one takes time and persistence, but pays long-term dividends.

Now that we know that we should eat more slowly and wisely, just *when* should we actually eat? For most people three meals a day are an accepted rule. Sometimes these are interspersed with snacks. This is a very good idea for active youngsters who burn a lot of energy. Milk and crackers or fruit juice and crackers offered between breakfast and lunch or lunch and dinner provide an energizing snack, which, if taken *midway* between meals, is unlikely to spoil the appetite for the next meal. The coffee break for adults could be desirable when indicated, but too often it is substituted for the good breakfast, which was bypassed. Breakfast is still the most important meal of the day!

Of prime importance to the performance of *all* family members is a good breakfast after the long night's fast. *All* is emphasized because repeatedly it has been found that a conscientious mother will see that her husband and children have an attractive, appetizing breakfast and neglect to eat it herself. Often this is because she thinks the omission will enable her to cut down on calories. Cut down on calories she may, but she also cuts out nutrients essential to her well-being.

A balanced, planned breakfast at home is likely to be more nutritious and less expensive than the empty calorie snacks available at the average snack bar. In general the stomach empties between three and one-half to four and one-half hours after a meal. It is then that you may experience hunger pangs. A carton of milk will do wonders to allay the sensation of hunger and not fill you up to the extent that you do not approach the next meal with zest.

Tea is another snack idea. A treat for your children, it is a relaxing way to visit with friends. A cup of tea makes you stop. It helps you get going again. Henry James, obviously a devotee of tea, once wrote, "There are few hours in life more agreeable than the hour dedicated to the ceremony known as afternoon tea."

It is a highly personal matter whether you eat three meals a day separated by five-to-six-hour intervals, or if you add between-meal snacks, or if you feel better eating small, more frequent meals. The stomach doesn't have a built-in clock, but through "sensation" often "tells time" to eat. You simply must find your own pattern.

Chapter 14

APPLE PIE FOR BREAKFAST? WHY NOT?

by Eloise R. Trescher, R.D.

Breakfast should be an event, not a brief encounter. Studies show that children's learning improves after starting the day with a good meal, and workers' productivity increases. Breakfast helps you to start the day with a sense of well-being, makes you alert, responsive. Without the first meal, it is possible but improbable that you will get your daily quota of the nutrients you require. Breakfast is your best beauty treatment. Have it in a relaxed way. Feed your body the nutrients it needs to supply energy for your early hours. The nutrients go through the digestive and the metabolic process at different rates and help to keep one's blood sugar sustained throughout the day. These nutrients—protein, fats, carbohydrates, minerals, vitamins, plus water—give you the balanced diet necessary to maintain you in good health.

Each nutrient plays an important role, sometimes several. Protein, minerals, and water build and repair worn-out tissues; carbohydrates, fats, and protein supply heat and energy; while water, minerals, and vitamins help regulate your body functions.

What is a good breakfast? Take your choice, anything you

like as long as it provides one-fourth to one-third of your day's requirements for calories and protein, and supplies some of the other essential nutrients.

A good breakfast for an average woman may consist of about 400 to 500 calories. The woman of reference on whom this theory is based is 5 feet 4 inches. The recommended calorie count for a healthy woman twenty-three to fifty years of age is approximately 2,000 calories a day. This, with a reasonable amount of physical activity, should keep her at her desired weight, not losing, nor gaining. When a woman is pregnant or lactating her needs are greater. As one grows older calorie needs are reduced. In general, 1,800 calories a day are sufficient for a woman from the age of fifty-one on, her energy needs decreasing as she becomes less active.

The man of the family should be with the family, too, at breakfast. Serve your husband a good breakfast, but keep in mind the man of reference is much taller and broader than you, and so needs proportionately more than you.

To start the day a good breakfast that gives you one-fourth of your necessary nutrients might be a serving of fruit or juice; an ounce of either meat, cheese, fish, or an egg; 2 slices of toast or a bowl of cereal (or 1 piece of toast and a smaller helping of cereal); ½ to 1 cup of milk; 1 level teaspoon of butter or margarine; 2 level teaspoons of jelly, jam, marmalade, or honey. You could use only 1 teaspoon of jam if you wanted a teaspoon of sugar in your coffee. Coffee and tea, alone, are free.

Apple pie for breakfast? Why not. Add a piece of cheese and even a small topping of ice cream, with a glass of milk. It may seem like a dessert to some, but to others it is a delicious breakfast. P.M. food in the A.M. is perfectly fine as long as you mix your nutrients and see that they keep good company.

A friend of mine has a sixteen-year-old son who has suddenly declared his independence at breakfast. He makes his own. His mother, in awe, told me a typical breakfast—orange juice, roast beef sandwich, hot oatmeal with milk, angel cake. Being a traditionalist, she worries about this unusual mixture. But this young man is practicing good nutrition. His breakfast includes protein, fats, calories, carbohydrates, minerals, and vitamins. Angel cake, for instance, is a good source of energy with egg whites, sugar, and flour. Children of all ages need calories for energy, and this boy is getting his share.

Serve breakfast with a flair, a matter of planning and priority. An attractive setting will lure your family to the table. After all, surprises are part of the fun. Set the table the night before. A mother should eat *with* her family, not afterward. Planning makes this possible. Being with them as a mother, not the cook, is important and makes cleaning up later that much easier and is time-saving for the mother.

If you are an early riser, set the stage then. While the coffee is percolating, perk up the table. Use lengths of bright-colored fabric (you only have to hem the ends) as tablecloths, or vary the setting with place mats, scoops of color. Change the scene often. Give variety to the eye as well as to the palate. In the center of the table put a fan of autumn leaves, a pumpkin, a pyramid of golden apples. A table set with imagination will help make breakfast a happy meal and not just a hasty one.

As you know, an adult should have 6 to 8 glasses of water a day, preferably between meals. If you drink 1 to 2 glasses on arising it will activate a quiet bowel and help promote a satisfactory bowel movement. Plan a regular time for this important part of your hygiene—about 20 minutes after breakfast is the best time. Constipation in a healthy individual is usually due to irregular habits and improper diet. If you experience unusual variation in your bowel habit, consult your doctor immediately.

Many mothers find it more relaxed and more comfortable to have the family come to the table in their robes. After a good breakfast allow enough time for hygiene and dressing. Having children organize their school work and books and clothes the night before will help avoid the morning scramble, the accompanying short tempers, which take away from energy gained from breakfast. And it's a good idea to keep all complaints and criticism away from the table. A positive atmosphere at breakfast will aid digestion whereas airing family differences will do just the opposite.

Breakfast may be small, medium, or large. But breakfast is for *every* member of the family *every* morning. Try cottage cheese or yoghurt with raspberries, blueberries, or stewed apricots. An alternative might be superb jam, such as Nantucket Beach Plum preserve or guava jelly—a splendid foil for the blandness of yoghurt. (No cooking here, please note, no pans to wash.) Protein and fruit are provided, and toast or crackers should be included. Protein is a natural for breakfast, a star starter to give energy. It also helps to offset hunger. Of Greek origin, "protein" means "of first importance."

Slice into an excellent source of double vitamins A and C, the cantaloupe. Wedge the top with slices of lemon and lime (both high in ascorbic acid). Small treats work large wonders at breakfast. Why not plan a week of breakfasts, giving them the same care you do to planning your weekly dinners? And post them in the kitchen as a reminder and encouragement to your family, giving them something to look forward to first thing in the morning.

A hearty cold breakfast could be a platter of thinly sliced ham and cheese—Cheddar, Swiss, caraway—with plenty of hot, crispy toast, crunchy rolls. Put all this on a lazy Susan and let everyone make his own, a smorgasbord breakfast. Have a variety of jams and jellies—ginger marmalade, Damson plum, blackberry, crab apple. Pitchers of juice and milk round out the meal. Afterward you can wrap up the ham and cheese not eaten for another easy, quick, nutritious breakfast.

Cocoa is a wonderful camouflage for milk. But this time try evaporated milk. This cocoa is different, and the children love it! You can make up large amounts, keep it in the refrigerator, and reheat for breakfast. (A child should have 3 to 4 cups of milk a day, adults, at least 2 cups.)

Cocoa

Ingredients
1/4 cup cocoa
1/3 cup sugar
1 3/4 cups water
13-ounce can evaporated milk

Method
In a saucepan mix thoroughly cocoa and sugar. Add water.
Bring to a boil. Add evaporated milk, and heat. Serve with a
dash of vanilla. Makes 3 generous cups.

When you're in a tizzy, and it's just one of those days, a
milkshake can take care of breakfast. It's quick, tastes good,
and provides everything a good breakfast should except
roughage and a relaxed atmosphere. Use a cup of milk with
fruit—ripe berries, a banana, or fresh or canned peaches, one
egg, and a scoop of vanilla ice cream or ice milk. Blend.
Pour into a tall glass (it will almost double in volume) and
serve.

On the weekends breakfast may be later and larger—
kidney stew and waffles, corn beef hash with poached egg,
scrapple with broiled apple rings, a galaxy of omelettes,
creamed chipped beef on English muffins. If you are looking
for a way to make a white sauce *without* butter, perhaps for
your chipped beef, try this:

White Sauce

Ingredients
2 level tablespoons flour
1 cup milk
Dash of paprika or few drops of yellow coloring
White pepper
Durkee's or McCormick Butter Salt

Method

Put flour in a saucepan; add milk gradually, smoothing out the lumps. Heat and stir constantly until thickened. At the end, add dash of paprika or few drops of yellow coloring, white pepper, and butter salt. Seves 3–4.

On a warm Saturday why not let the children have a breakfast picnic? Into a bandana handkerchief put a leg of cold chicken, carrot sticks, some bread with honey. Fill canteens with milk and fruit juice. It's easy; it's nutritious; it's fun; it's a change.

If anyone in your family has to avoid cholesterol, "Egg Beaters," and "Second Nature," frozen egg mixtures, are cholesterol-free. Use them for scrambled eggs, in waffles and pancakes. They are delicious and if you don't tell, no one will know the difference.

An alternate mixture might be made at home. For one person, use the whites of 3 eggs, 2 level tablespoons nonfat dry milk, 3 drops yellow color. Limiting the amount of cholesterol for the entire family is prudent and good health insurance.

Chapter 15

LUNCH—THE GREAT ENERGIZER

by Eloise R. Trescher, R.D.

The middle of everyone's day should be punctuated by a well-balanced lunch, a delicious hyphen that both connects and separates a full daily schedule. Lunch is a signal to stop, to revive flagging energies, to make you more alert for the rest of the day. It provides time for a change of pace, to relax and socialize, a time to refuel for afternoon activities. Everyone should count on lunch, as it should furnish about one-third of one's daily food requirements—the calories, protein, and other essential nutrients one needs to build and maintain a strong, healthy body. When you come back from lunch, whether it be from the next room or the restaurant across town, you often come back with a new slant for the whole afternoon.

Many individuals, both adults and children, muddle through the day in a twilight of awareness, fatigued and listless, just because of poor eating habits. Their day drags. What they should realize is that a nutritious lunch is a center way station, and one that should include selections from the four food groups. It is best to include all four, but not eat too much of any.

The four food groups: Milk and milk products; vegetables and fruit; meat, fish, poultry, eggs, and cheese; bread and cereals, whole grain or enriched.

A friend who usually eats lunch at home alternates her patterns. If she is at a desk or a sewing table most of the morning, she eats her lunch walking around the house or her garden. If she has had a very active morning, she lunches peacefully on a card table she has placed by the sunniest window in the living room. When possible, no matter what the season, she packs a picnic for her executive husband who she thinks is too desk-bound. Together they picnic in a park, overlooking a pier, sometimes the zoo. One time she even dragged her china, the lunch, and her husband to an abandoned boxcar. "I'll do almost anything to take his mind off his work at lunch," she says. And there are three subjects, she claims, you must never discuss at lunch—children, money, or business.

Sandwiches, open or closed, have always been old faithfuls at lunchtime. Try vegetables to add a new twist, zest, and variety to this usual lunch menu. Chop or grate leftover cooked or raw vegetables and mix them with mayonnaise. This makes a delicious spread for meat or chicken sandwiches and is marvelous in salad mixtures such as egg, tuna, chopped liver, or chicken. You can concoct all sorts of vegetable combinations depending on your imagination and ingenuity, plus your knowledge of your family's avowed hates and preferences. Vegetables are all to the good, as they contain minerals and vitamins and provide bulk and residue.

To use as a mix with mayonnaise, chop raw vegetables such as celery, carrots, onions, zucchini, broccoli, spinach, watercress, cauliflower, green peppers, parsley, tomatoes, cucumbers. Chopped cooked vegetables that combine well with meat or chicken sandwiches are string beans, stewed tomatoes, and carrots. And instead of lettuce, why not try cole slaw or sauerkraut?

Lunch is an exercise in good taste and good nutrition that should be part of every day. Lunch at home or in a restaurant is your own free choice, but it is often the lunch parties at a club or at someone's house that sometimes take grace and a certain strategy to avoid overeating. When served an abundance—too much chicken salad, too many spiced peaches—learn to nibble. Learn how to eat slowly. When offered seconds, take small portions. The gesture will be observed (but rarely the amount) and your hostess will feel complimented. This is the time to be a scintillating conversationalist. Address yourself to the company rather than to the food. Soon your plate will be whisked away when you're half finished. This is a good way to cut down on calories without attracting attention to yourself.

No matter where you have lunch, home or away, the four food groups should be served. Have that cheeseburger at the corner drugstore, but start off with a glass of tomato juice or V-8 juice. For dessert choose some fruit or ice cream, and milk, coffee, or tea—a simple lunch but a sound one.

With the scarcity of help and demands on one's time, a lunch that can be prepared quickly is always welcome. Here, a spur-of-the-moment lunch including the vegetable, often the forgotten food at lunchtime:

Curried tomato-and-chicken bouillon
Open-face sandwich
Fruit bowl
Coffee, tea, or milk

To make the curried tomato-and-chicken bouillon soup, combine equal parts of tomato juice and chicken bouillon. Add a generous dash of curry powder and serve hot.

For your open-face sandwich arrange bread slices or halved English muffins on a shallow pan. Spread with a film of butter or margarine. Cover each with asparagus tips, chopped spinach, lightly cooked broccoli, or mushrooms. Place sliced or chopped turkey, chicken, ham, tuna, shrimp, lobster, crab, or deviled eggs on the chosen vegetable. Top with Swiss cheese or mayonnaise, and sprinkle with paprika. Broil the sandwiches or bake them at 375° until hot (about 10 minutes). The fruit bowl dessert might be any one or a mixture of these fruits—polished apples, bananas, Tokay grapes, and tangerines.

For children who say they won't eat vegetables, including them surreptitiously in sandwiches is a pleasant surprise and is one way to teach them to eat a food that they might otherwise refuse. If they catch you chopping, just say, "Joe Namath likes his sandwiches this way." If children are taught to eat properly at home, they will eat properly at school. And it is a lot easier to build good food habits than to correct poor ones.

Nutritious school lunches are vital to your child's activity, attention span, and learning ability. Any child will eat what he likes five days straight, but soon he'll tire even of his favorites. It is up to the mother and school nutritionist to add variety to well-balanced meals. Surprises often ease the traffic in food trading. Children who bargain and barter away their lunches end up with poorly balanced meals, not only for themselves, but also for others. Given an attractive meal, chances are they'll want to keep it.

Important to any bag lunch is a broad-mouthed thermos. It will keep tuna salad cold and your child can eat his lunch right out of the thermos. Send a supply of straws to school too. Most children will drink almost anything if it can be sipped through a straw. At home, the wise mother keeps a generous supply of straws within easy reach for soups, juices, and milk drinks.

For an alive and vivacious family, plan and serve tempting nutritious meals. They deserve top priority. A lunch you might send to school which has child appeal could be:

Baked bean and chopped ham sandwich
Celery sticks stuffed with soft cheese
Candy apple on a stick
Thermos of a favorite cream soup or milk
Ginger cookies

To make the baked bean and chopped ham sandwich,

spread the bread with tomato paste and mustard, and add onion, baked beans, and thinly sliced cooked, leftover chopped ham or leftover hot dogs.

With children in school, a small winter lunch at home is a friendly afternoon. I like this broccoli soufflé, as it incorporates one of the best green vegetables, which is rich in both vitamins A and C when cooked:

Broccoli Soufflé

Ingredients
3 tablespoons butter or margarine
3 tablespoons flour
1 cup milk
3 large eggs, separated
1/4 teaspoon salt
1/8 teaspoon pepper
1 cup finely chopped, well-drained cooked broccoli

Method
In a saucepan over low heat melt the butter. Stir in flour. Add the milk; cook and stir constantly over moderately low heat; heat until thickened and bubbly.

Remove from heat. Gradually and vigorously stir into slightly beaten egg yolks. Mix in salt, pepper, and broccoli. Beat egg whites until they hold slightly tipping peaks. Fold in broccoli mixture.

Turn into an ungreased 1-quart soufflé dish. Bake in a slow 350° oven, 45 minutes. Serve at once.

Chapter 16

DINNER—OUR MOST SOCIAL OF ALL MEALS

by Eloise R. Trescher, R.D.

In Medieval England, "dynner" was a study in manners, a play of protocol. A man knew his rank, a man knew where he sat by the salt—the all-important salt, the first container always placed on the table. Spoons were provided by the host, but each man brought his own knife. And the food was a nutritious feast from "lambe boyled to larkes to quinces and pippins."

Today dinner is *still* our most social of all meals. And even though it may be simple fare, it is our most congenial gathering. More than a scene of protocol, it is a practical setting. It is the meal when we are able to be together again with our family, or perhaps a reunion with friends, a time to relax, the day's work done.

A well-planned dinner *completes* our nutrition quota for the day. At every meal you should receive one third of your nutrients—the protein, fats, carbohydrates, minerals, vitamins, and water that you need for a balanced diet, a healthy life. You should never forget breakfast, nor neglect lunch, but if you happen to slip up during the day, dinner can fill in, in part, but never fully.

A hungry man certainly doesn't go to bed happy. A good,

nutritious, satisfying dinner helps to pave the way to a restful night's sleep—and other healthy pleasures en route to the arms of Morpheus. You wake to a better day.

Dinner should be enjoyed for its own sake, rather than accompanying something considered to be more important. If you're going to watch television, do it around the clock if you like, but not around the dinner table. Dinner should be a relaxed, pleasant time for each person, beginning with the youngest member of the family. It should be a time for happy discussions, what one has seen, learned, an amusing experience, an interesting event at school or at work. It could be the one time for family forums, planning a vacation, the news of the world, yours and others'. You should count on conversation as often as you count calories.

It is not the time for lectures, nor mention of problems, nor poor behavior. These should be dealt with at another time, but never at mealtime. Perhaps you might even let your young son wear his new baseball cap once or twice. It will certainly surprise him, and it won't be anything new. In 1664, Samuel Pepys, the chronicler of London, wrote that he "caught a strange cold in my head by flinging off my hat at dinner."

With children getting home from school at all hours, and hungry, a preliminary snack might be available on arrival, such as a substantial soup, a good salad—antipasto with crackers—or a milkshake. Such offerings would hopefully tide youngsters over until Dad arrives. For children who have schoolwork, dinner should be at an early hour. Adult martinis aren't as important as those children's marks in school. At least not to the children.

Dinner, as well as every meal, should include the four food groups—(1) meat, fish, poultry, eggs, and cheese; (2) vegetables and fruits; (3) milk and milk products; (4) bread and cereals. I recently heard of a family that has meat loaf and broccoli, even lasagna, at their first meal of the day. Radically changing their eating pattern, they have their dinner at breakfast.

The father of this active family decided they could never get a quorum at night with everyone going off in different directions at different times. Besides, he and his wife wanted to see their five children. Dinner at breakfast is certainly an innovation, a brave move, and not many mothers would have the stamina to do it, and the spunk to say "dinner is served" at 6:50 A.M., but it is nutritionally sound and has made this family closer together. Their meal in the evening is a buffet of cheese and crackers and an enormous salad, with everyone eating when and whatever he likes.

Many casseroles, easily prepared and leisurely enjoyed, include all four food groups, and every one includes at least two and often three groups. Here are two casseroles I like, not only for their flavor, but also for the balance of ingredients:

Pork Chops Nantucket

Ingredients
4 loin pork chops, 1 inch thick
4 thick slices Bermuda or Spanish onion
1 20-ounce can tomato wedges
4 tablespoons long grain or wild rice (uncooked)
Salt and pepper to taste

Method
Dredge pork chops in seasoned flour and brown on both sides in a minimum of oil. Pour off excess fat. Arrange chops in a casserole. Place a thick slice of onion on each chop. Add tomatoes including juice. Place 1 tablespoon of rice on each chop. Cover casserole and bake at 350° for 1 hour, 12 minutes (approximately). Time varies depending upon the thickness of the chops. Pleasant variations in seasoning are rosemary, marjoram, or thyme. If additional moisture is needed, tomato juice or beef bouillon may be added. Serves 4.

Crab Imperial Superb

Ingredients
1 green pepper, finely diced
2 pimientos, chopped
1 tablespoon English mustard
1 tablespoon salt
1/2 teaspoon white pepper
2 eggs
1 cup mayonnaise
3 pounds lump (backfin) crab meat, well picked

Method
Mix all ingredients except crab. Add crab meat and mix well with fingers to prevent breaking crab lumps. Place mixture in individual shells. Top with a light coating of mayonnaise and sprinkle with paprika. Bake at 350° for 15 minutes or until mayonnaise browns. Serve hot or cold. Serves 9 to 12.

Crusty rolls, a salad, and dessert, with coffee, tea, or milk served with either of these two casseroles round out the meal. Another casserole, a carrot pudding, as a vegetable, might be a new treat for your family, and spring carrots are filled with vitamins, especially vitamin A.

Mrs. Keyser's Carrot Pudding

Ingredients
10 medium-sized carrots
1/2 green pepper, finely cut
2 tablespoons grated onion
2 tablespoons butter
1 tablespoon flour
1 tablespoon sugar
1 cup hot milk
Salt and pepper to taste

Method

Cook carrots until tender; drain and press in a food mill. Sauté grated onion and green pepper in butter until onion is golden brown. Stir in flour, sugar, and salt and pepper to taste. Add gradually the cup of hot milk and keep stirring until sauce slightly thickens. Combine with carrot purée and turn into a buttered casserole. Cover top with bread crumbs, dot with butter, and bake 30 minutes in a 350° oven. Serves 4 to 6.

Colette once wrote that when she was thirsty she drank water, when she was hungry she drank wine. More and more Americans, perhaps because of travel and taste, are drinking more and more wine, especially at dinner. And so when discussing dinner I feel we should consider the calorie count of wine. Whether it is red or white hasn't anything to do with it; it's whether it is a dry or sweet wine. The calorie range of wine goes from 75 to 165 calories per 3 1/3 ounces, a scant half cup. In general, the dry wines such as Chablis, Burgundy, or dry champagne have from 75 to 100 calories to that scant half cup. Sherry, port, vermouth, a sweet champagne, are higher, ranging from 100 to 165 calories.

The calorie value of distilled liquors such as rye, scotch, bourbon, gin, rum, vodka, and brandy is from 75 calories to 100 calories per 1 ounce, depending on proof. Of course, with both wine, fermented, and liquors, distilled, it all depends on the quantity you imbibe.

Dinner for the family at least one night a week should be especially festive. Make it a small celebration. Have the soup or dessert in the living room. When you change courses why not rooms? Or another evening you might put a table by an open fire—one card table or two put together. You can buy round tabletops that fold away neatly for storage. A round table is cozy and conducive to conversation and an enjoyable meal. Any room can be a room to dine in. One evening I remember happily, was a dinner in an unfinished room, actually a bedroom, of an old house of a young couple. Walls were exposed, saw horses supported wonderful plank tables, and the scaffolding made a sculptural background. It was original and fun.

As for Sunday dinners, they may just be the time to teach your son or daughter how to carve. This is fast becoming a lost art with the young. Yet a good carver is always a welcome guest. Lord Chesterfield, who always had a lot to say to his son in letters, once wrote to his offspring: "Have you learned to carve? Do you use yourself to carve adroitly and genteely, without hacking half an hour across a bone . . . and without overturning the glasses into your neighbors' pockets?" When dinner is served, having the children help makes more than a meal, it makes for good company.

A well-thought-out, nutritious dinner is a unifying climax to a busy day, a perfect ending if you take time to plan it that way.

Chapter 17

NUTRITION FOR A TEENAGE ATHLETE

by Eloise R. Trescher, R.D.

Coaches can counsel, but it's the mothers who serve. And for teenage athletes a subtle training table at home all year long with nutritious, well-balanced meals will produce the winning teams. Not the crash diets for wrestlers, nor the seasonal stuffing of football players, but instead, good sound strategy in food selection, year in and year out from birth on, is the best preparation to insure superior athletic performance.

Good nutrition scores innumerable points for teenage athletes. It sustains endurance in short- and long-term events, controls body weight, promotes muscle tone, clear skin, and mental alertness. It also helps prevent dental cavities and improves learning ability, coordination, agility, flexibility, strength, vigor, posture, control, and speed of action.

The body must be supplied with the right nutrients in sufficient amounts if it is to grow and develop. This is especially true the first twenty years of life. Teenage boys need more calories and more of almost every nutrient except iron than girls of the same age. Teenage girls need the iron to manufacture new blood. A nutritionally balanced diet helps to build strong, healthy bodies.

Boys are usually better nourished than girls simply because

they eat more. The pencil-slim silhouette most teenage girls want often stands in the way of their proper eating. Yet, you build your figure yourself, and it should be done with knowledge, not fads. If you prepare early, there'll be no need for redesigning later on.

Most teenagers admire their athletes, striving to be like them, following their examples. And good nutrition is one of the better examples to follow, contributing to youths' effectiveness, purpose, and enthusiasm.

What one eats 48 hours before either a short- or long-term event is important. In that period before competition, it is advisable to reduce food residue. The athlete should avoid raw fruits, raw vegetables (except lettuce), vegetables with seeds, whole grain products, relishes, popcorn, nuts, jams, preserves, and gravy. Instead he should choose cooked fruit and vegetables, fruit and vegetable juices (except prune juice), skim milk, enriched bread, rice, noodles, spaghetti, potatoes without skins, macaroni, roasted and broiled meats, poultry, fish, cheese, eggs (only 3 a week), jellies, honey, and syrups.

The pre-event meal should precede the competition by 3 to 4 hours. This allows time for digestion and absorption of the meal, and it is not too long a period to allow feelings of hunger to develop. A mother might serve this menu as a pre-event meal, remembering to salt food well:

1 serving of roasted or broiled meat or poultry
1 serving of mashed potatoes or one baked potato without skin, or 1/2 cup macaroni, noodles, or rice
1 serving of vegetables
1 cup of skim milk
1 teaspoon of butter or margarine and 2 teaspoons of jelly or other sweets
1 serving of fruit
Sugar cookies or plain cake
1–2 cups of extra beverage

Fruit juice in small amounts is far better as a source of

energy for pre-event snacks than honey or sugar, as it supplies both carbohydrates and fluid. Fruit juice is an energy giver for anyone, at any time.

Much of what one is to be—one's strength, one's physique, one's endurance—begins when one is conceived. The kind and amount of food the mother eats during pregnancy has a direct influence on her offspring. If a child is properly fed until the age of two, the foods to be included in a well-balanced diet are the same throughout life, the amounts vary depending upon height, age, sex, and activity.

Eating habits and attitudes we form as children often decide what we eat as adults. Adults should not openly talk about a child's eating problems or dislike for a certain food, say cucumbers, as it might influence his eating habits. A child quickly learns that he can upset his parents in the way he acts toward his food. This, unfortunately, can continue through teenage years. A thin child often likes to remain thin because of the attention gained from his parents. The same is true for the fatter child.

Good nutrition is not a mystery, but it is a well-planned detective story, finding the right clues, the culprits (not the butler in the library, but perhaps too much butter in the kitchen). The best lead is to employ a wide variety in the selection of foods that are to be included in moderation in daily menus.

The following foods in the amounts listed are essential to the well-balanced daily diet for average teenagers:

Milk—4 cups (may include that used in cooking or food preparation)

Meat, fish, poultry, cheese, eggs—a total of 5 to 7 ounces (limit eggs to 3 a week)

Dark green or deep yellow vegetables—1/2 cup

Citrus fruit or juice, cantaloupe, or strawberries—1 serving

Other vegetables and fruit—2 servings or 1 cup

Bread and cereal, whole grain, enriched (or potato)—13 to 14 servings

Fat, margarine, butter, mayonnaise, other fat spreads—10 teaspoons

Note: Additional foods may be necessary for some individuals or youngsters in order for them to maintain correct weight.

This is approximately 2,500 calories, taking care of protein, mineral, and vitamin allowances for teenagers. A training table for the teenage athlete is good for the whole family. The chief difference between the ultimate diet for the athlete and his more sedentary brother is a matter of calories. A teenage athlete who is exercising strenuously may need 3,000 or more calories daily, while an adult woman needs only about 1,700 to 2,000, and an adult man about 2,400 to 2,700. (Calorie allowances for healthy adults cover ages twenty-three on.)

Snacks are part of any teenager's lifestyle. They particularly like finger food, out-of-the-hand snacks. It is a good idea to set aside an open shelf in the refrigerator especially for a teenager and his friends—nothing forbidden—provided whatever they eat or drink doesn't spoil their appetite for the next meal or effect an undesirable gain in weight.

Some good, tasty, nutritious snacks could be cheese, cottage cheese, milk, fruit juices, milk soups, milk shakes, cocoa made with milk, custard, ice cream, ice milk, sandwiches, cookies, crackers, tomato juice, V-8 juice, dried fruits (such as raisins, peaches, apricots, and prunes), apples, fresh fruit, cereal with milk, leftovers, peanut butter, raw vegetables (such as celery, carrots, cauliflower, zucchini, cucumbers, tomatoes, turnips, cabbage, radishes) popcorn, nuts.

You might include some pitchers of juices on that open shelf—lemonade, limeade, orange juice, pineapple juice, apricot juice, apple juice, grape juice, or cranberry juice.

For a gathering after the game, teenagers particularly like "Flora's Moremore," a nutritious casserole parents will probably borrow for their own:

Flora's Moremore

Ingredients
1/2-pound box spaghetti
1/4 cup oil
1 large onion, sliced
1 clove garlic
1 green pepper, sliced
1 #2 can tomatoes
2 cans tomato paste and 2 cans water
1 bay leaf
1 teaspoon oregano
2 pounds ground beef rolled into small balls
1 pound sharp American cheese, grated
Salt and pepper to taste

Method
Boil spaghetti 12 minutes and blanch by pouring cold water over it. Drain. To make the sauce: Heat oil in skillet, sauté onion, garlic, and pepper, add tomatoes, tomato paste, 2 cans water, bay leaf, and oregano. Salt and pepper to taste, add beef balls and cook until tender, about 10 minutes. Grease a 3-quart casserole. Put one layer of spaghetti on the bottom, then a layer of sauce, next a layer of grated cheese on top. Bake about 45 minutes in a 350° oven. Serve hot. Serves about 18. This, with a tossed salad and French bread, is a full and delicious meal.

A sweet, simple dessert for teenagers is angel cake with variations. Cut an angel cake into three or more horizontal layers. Spread each layer with partially thawed frozen raspberries, strawberries, or peaches. Frost the outside with lightly sweetened sour or whipped cream. Of if you prefer an ice-cream cake, put softened ice cream between layers, and then put into freezer. For a tasty addition, for adult only, sprinkle rum over the ice-cream cake before putting it into the freezer.

Chapter 18

VITAMINS—FOR YOUR VERY LIFE

by Eloise R. Trescher, R.D.

VITAL VITAMIN STATISTICS

Every known vitamin of today has had a mysterious past, always elusive. However, many of the mysteries have been solved by dedicated scientists in constant search. Take vitamin C, the now familiar ascorbic acid. Although only identified in 1928, its history goes back almost 400 years. Without vitamin C, Jacques Cartier might never have colonized Newfoundland; without vitamin C, Admiral Nelson might never have conquered the fleet of Napoleon.

In 1535 with 100 of his 110 men sick with scurvy, Cartier gave his expedition an Indian recipe of "spruce pine needle soup," rich in vitamin C. Within six days his men were cured. Some 200 years later, James Lind, Physician to the Royal Navy, started a daily ration of "two oranges and one lemon" for seamen suffering from scurvy. They too recovered and by the time of the Napoleonic Wars the Royal Navy's fighting force was doubled, chiefly because of a daily dose of fresh citrus juice. "Lind," it is said, "as much as Nelson broke the power of Napoleon."

History, so it seems, was helped by vitamin C. Yet vitamin

C, as well as the others, was identified and isolated in the twentieth century, our century. One needs the knowledge of the chemist, the biochemist, the physiologist, the pathologist, and the clinician to fully understand the interaction of these vitamins and the role they play in the availability and utilization of other nutrients. Every day the mystery is being unfolded gradually by researchers in laboratories throughout the world.

Much has been discovered, but there is much that is unknown. One important fact is that vitamin pills or capsules are *not* substitutes for food. They contain only the *known* or discovered vitamins. Food contains *both* the discovered and undiscovered.

The vitamins we are concerned with and considering in this chapter are those for which Recommended Dietary Allowances (RDA) have been made by the Food and Nutrition Board, National Academy of Sciences, National Research Council. They are vitamins A, D, E, and ascorbic acid, and vitamins of the B complex, folacin, niacin, riboflavin, thiamin, B_6, and B_{12}.

All the vitamins that the healthy individual needs are present in food. By choosing food from each of the four food groups, you are assured of adequate amounts of vitamins as well as minerals and protein.

FOUR FOOD GROUPS

• The meat group supplies you with thiamin, riboflavin, niacin, B_6 and B_{12}, vitamin A (only in liver and egg yolk).
• The milk group gives significant amounts of all vitamins except vitamin C and thiamin. It is an excellent source of riboflavin.
• Fruits and vegetables are suppliers of vitamins A and C.
• Breads and cereals, whole grain and enriched, are good sources of thiamin, riboflavin, and niacin.

The word "vitamin" comes from the Latin *vita*, meaning

life. And once you realize the benefits gained from each vitamin, the name seems indeed appropriate. Your family doctor, not TV nor cardboard advertising drugstores, is the one to tell you when you may need additional vitamins prescribed by pill, capsule, or injection. And although each vitamin plays a specific role in the prevention of specific diseases, their effectiveness is enhanced when they play in concert with other nutrients.

To truly appreciate vitamins, you should know *what* vitamins do for you. With well-balanced, nutritious meals they can easily be part of your life.

There are two kinds of vitamins. One group of vitamins— A, D, and E—are called fat-soluble and are stored by the body. Ascorbic acid and the vitamins of the B complex are called water-soluble and are not stored to any great extent in the body. These vitamins are easily lost through heat, oxidation, and "leeching," or soaking out in water. Citrus juices and tomato juice should be stored in a covered container in the refrigerator. Foods should be cooked only a short time and in as little water as possible in order to preserve vitamins of the B complex and ascorbic acid. Water is not a food, but it is essential to carry nutrients to the various cells within the body and to carry away waste products.

Vitamin A is essential in maintaining the normal ability of the eye to see in the darkness, light and dark adaptation, as when entering a movie theatre. It also promotes healthy skin and mucous membranes, and helps bone growth. An excess of vitamin A in children can stop growth, and bones become fragile. In older people an excess can result in loss of appetite as well as of hair.

Vitamin D helps in the calcification of bones and aids absorption of calcium from food in the digestive tract. Bone deformities occur when you haven't enough vitamin D, as in rickets. Excess vitamin D can also be harmful, causing bone softening, loss of appetite, calcification of kidneys, and eventually kidney failure. Massive doses of vitamins A and D are known to be toxic and should be taken only on a physician's prescription.

Ascorbic acid, the conqueror of scurvy, maintains in a normal state the "ground substance" in which tissue cells are embedded and cemented together. Ascorbic acid also promotes firm blood vessel walls and contributes to normal healing of wounds and bones.

Niacin helps keep your nervous system healthy as well as your skin, mouth, tongue, and digestive tract. It also enables cells to use other nutrients. A niacin deficiency induces the disease pellagra, a name given by Italian scientists meaning "rough skin." The skin becomes red; the tongue is irritated; and in extreme deficiency, insanity and death can result. Pellagra still prevails in part of the world, but to a limited extent.

Riboflavin enables blood cells to use oxygen and contributes to the health of your tongue, skin, lips, and eyes.

Thiamin helps give you a normal appetite and digestion, keeps your nervous system healthy, and prevents irritability. It is also necessary in helping the body make available energy from food. Beriberi is caused by a deficiency of thiamin.

Vitamin B_6 plays a major role in amino acid metabolism, as well as in red cell regeneration. Without vitamin B_6 you do not form antibodies normally. It is another vitamin that helps your nervous system function as it should.

Vitamin B_{12} is important to your protein, fat, and carbohydrate metabolism, helps bone marrow cells, as well as your nervous system. It also protects you against pernicious anemia.

Vitamin E is necessary in small amounts in human nutrition.

The widespread interest in this vitamin is due to the misinterpretation of the results of research on experimental animals. Vitamin E is present in a wide variety of foods, and for those who have a varied well-balanced diet, a deficiency is highly unlikely. In lower animals it does play a role in reproduction, but in man its more important role is protecting vitamin A.

Dr. E. V. McCollum, discoverer of vitamins A and D, was chairman of the biochemistry department of the School of Hygiene and Public Health at the Johns Hopkins University when I was director of the Nutrition Clinic. Whenever I had a problem I could go to him. One of his dicta was "the right kind of food is the most important single factor in promoting health."

Certain foods contain certain vitamins; often they contain more than one. Vitamin A is found in all deep-green- and deep-yellow-colored foods. Listed here, a choice of vitamin A's vegetables and fruits:

beet greens	chives *	escarole
broccoli *	collards *	garden cress
carrots	dandelion greens *	green tops of
chard	dock *	spring onions *
chicory greens	tomatoes *	kale
lamb quarters *	sweet potatoes	peaches (yellow
mustard greens *	turnip greens	fleshed)
parsley	watercress *	mangoes *
peppers, red *	winter squash	papaya *
poke shoots	apricots	pitanga (Surinam
pumpkin	cantaloupe *	cherry)
spinach *		plums, purple

There are very few sources of vitamin A in the animal kingdom compared to vegetables and fruits. The richest

* Indicates good sources of ascorbic acid as well, if eaten raw, steamed, or cooked a short time in a small amount of water.

source of vitamin A in all kingdoms, however, is liver—all kinds. It is surpassed only by fish liver oils. Liver is not a popular food, and if it were, there wouldn't be enough to go around. Egg yolk, whole milk, fortified skim milk, buttermilk, butter, cream, cheese (except cottage), and ice cream all contain vitamin A. Other animal sources, some of them used frequently, are weakfish, swordfish, squid, crab, and other fish such as blue, rock, and king.

Vitamin C foods are oranges, grapefruit, cantaloupe, tomatoes, lemons, limes, tangerines, strawberries, potatoes, cauliflower, green peppers, and cabbage. Also those vegetables and fruits marked with an asterisk in the vitamin A group.

The American diet is most likely to be deficient in vitamin A and ascorbic acid. Vitamins of the B complex are so well distributed if one chooses one's meals from the four food groups, there is little likelihood of a deficiency. The chief source of vitamin D is sunlight. Remember, though, the ultraviolet rays do not pass through ordinary window glass, so you have to get out in the sun to get your vitamin D. Foods containing this vitamin are fish liver oils and vitamin D milk.

No one food can supply you with every vitamin. Yet there is a wide range, a delicious variety. It's up to you to choose wisely. Food comes in all colors, all flavors, all vitamins. Enjoy it.

Chapter 19

PROTEIN POWER

by Eloise R. Trescher, R.D.

You simply cannot live without protein. It is different from all other kinds of food substances in that it contains the nitrogen that is necessary for life. Named by the Greeks, "protein" means "first importance," and indeed it is. In the United States there is no shortage of protein, but in many underdeveloped countries children sicken and die for lack of it.

You need protein to grow and to repair the wear and tear that is constantly going on in body tissues. Proteins are structural elements, the principal part of the many fibers of connective tissue—collagenous, reticular (or netlike), and elastic. And this is just the beginning of the vast role proteins play. As enzymes, their functions are numerous and impressive. For example, certain muscle proteins are involved in converting chemical energy into mechanical work.

As intra-membrane carriers, proteins serve as shuttles in the transport of molecules and ions across cell membranes. Proteins also provide a carrier function in plasma, the fluid portion of the blood in which the corpuscles are suspended. Antibody proteins help protect the body's defense against infections. And as hormonal messengers, such as growth hormone and insulin, proteins carry information that regulates cell permeability and metabolism. Proteins furnish a source of fixed nitrogen for the synthesis of certain basic substances. Heme, for example, a deep-red pigment, is a constituent of hemoglobin. Protein may also serve as a source of energy.

Now that we know the myriad functions protein performs for us, just how much protein do we need? All through life, protein is an essential nutrient, but infants, children, adolescents, pregnant and lactating women have special protein requirements for growth. The chart on page 156 of Daily Recommended Dietary Allowances was designed by the Food and Nutrition Board, National Academy of Sciences, National Research Council.

Proteins exist in both the animal and vegetable kingdoms. Amino acids linked together in a chain form the main structure of proteins. The quality of the protein is determined by *which* amino acids are used, how often they are repeated in the chain, and the order in which they are joined. There are 200 or more amino acids, but for humans we may divide them into two groups—the dispensable, or nonessential, and the indispensable, or essential. The indispensable amino acids must be obtained from our food. The human body can synthesize the nonessential.

There are eight indispensable amino acids for the adult, and all can be found in meat, fish, poultry, eggs, milk, and cheese. The eight are: isoleucine, leucine, lysine, methionine (cystine), phenylalanine (tyrosine), threonine, tryptophan, valine. A ninth, histidine, is necessary for infants.

Roots, nuts, fruits, tubers, legumes, and cereals may lack one or more the indispensable amino acids, but the deficiency may be supplemented by eating a food from each of the two groups *at the same time*. A common example is cereal and milk. Cereal and milk are a good combination any time, and a favorite bedtime snack for many. It is vital to remember that the time factor, the togetherness of each group, is essential in protein synthesis.

We know what protein does for our bodies and how much we need to keep ourselves in health, but where do we get it? The chart on page 157 of certain selected foods will help you add up your daily protein allowance. Keep it handy when you're planning your family meals.

It is important to remember that when calorie intake is

reduced, the efficiency of protein utilization is decreased. Think about this the next time you go on a diet budgeting calories. When energy intake is impaired by restriction of calories or illness caused by infection, fever, or surgical trauma, special effort must be made to ensure an adequate intake of both energy and protein. Rather than that old cliché, "feed a cold and starve a fever," you should feed both the cold and the fever. As your temperature goes up, more energy is used, so you should increase your calories by eating wisely.

A second erroneous belief is that muscular work increases the need for protein. Studies indicate that a small increase is needed for the *development* of muscles *during conditioning.* However, when this is accomplished no increment need be added for work. For healthy people, there is little evidence that exceeding the recommended allowance for protein is either beneficial or harmful.

Most Americans eat more than they really need, and far more protein than they need. Ours is a protein-oriented culture, from peanut butter to pork chops.

For a family dinner or a party supper, here are two recipes that provide both protein and a bit of variety. Both can be prepared in advance.

Mrs. Gott's Bran Muffins

Ingredients
2 cups 100% Nabisco Bran
2 cups boiling water
3 cups sugar
1 cup shortening
4 eggs
5 cups flour
5 teaspoons baking soda
1 teaspoon salt
1 quart buttermilk
4 cups Kellogg's All-Bran

Method

Combine Nabisco Bran with boiling water, then cool. Cream sugar with shortening. Add the eggs, one at a time, to the creamed mixture, beating well. Sift flour with baking soda and salt and mix alternately with buttermilk. Then combine with cooled Bran mixture and creamed mixture. Add the All Bran and stir well. Bake at 400° for 15 minutes in greased muffin tins. If using small muffin tins, check after 12 minutes. This batter may be halved for smaller amounts. It keeps well, covered, in the refrigerator for up to 2 weeks. Bake as needed.

Mrs. Lawrence Harper's Almond Pudding

Ingredients
1 cup roasted almonds, unblanched
1/2 cup shortening
1/2 cup granulated sugar
1 egg yolk
1/2 teaspoon almond extract
1/4 cup milk
1 cup sifted flour
2 teaspoons baking powder
1/2 teaspoon salt

Topping
1 egg white
3 tablespoons honey
1 tablespoon butter
1/4 cup granulated sugar

Method

Chop almonds fine. Cream shortening and sugar. Beat in egg yolk and almond extract. Stir in milk and almonds. Sift flour, baking powder, and salt; add to cream mixture. Spread in bottom of greased baking pan (10-by-10-by-1-inch). Combine topping ingredients; beat well, pour over batter, and sprinkle with sugar. Bake 15 minutes at 400° oven. Serve hot or cold with cream.

The two menus below show two different ways you can come up to the required protein allowance if you feel you might not be eating enough protein. Both, you will notice, exceed the recommended allowance. Both menus include the four food groups. These menus demonstrate how easy it is to put protein in your daily diet.

Plenty-of-protein Menus

With meat:	AMOUNT	PROTEIN GRAMS
BREAKFAST		
fruit or juice	1 serving	1
broiled ham	2 ounces	14
pancakes	2	4
		19
LUNCH		
tomato juice	1 cup	2
roast beef sandwich:		
enriched white bread	2 slices	4
roast beef	2 ounces	14
lettuce and mayonnaise	—	· trace
milk	1 cup	9
banana	1 large	1
		30
DINNER		
broiled fish	4 ounces	28
mashed potato with milk	1 cup	4
Harvard beets	½ cup	1
spinach and watercress salad	1 serving	1
Thousand Island dressing	2 tablespoons	trace
fresh fruit compote	1 serving	1
cookies	1	1
		36
	Total: 85 grams of protein	
Meatless:	AMOUNT	PROTEIN GRAMS
BREAKFAST		
fruit or juice	1 serving	1
oatmeal, cooked	1 cup	5
milk	1 cup	9
muffin	1	3
		18

Meatless:	AMOUNT	PROTEIN GRAMS
LUNCH		
peanut butter, lettuce and tomato sandwich		
enriched white bread	2 slices	4
peanut butter	2 tablespoons	8
lettuce	1-2 leaves	—
tomato	3-4 slices	1
milk	1 cup	9
apple pie	1 section	3
		25
DINNER		
baked beans	¾ cup	12
Boston brown bread	1 slice	3
broccoli	½ cup	3
lettuce hearts,	1/6th head	—
roquefort dressing	½ ounce	3
fresh strawberries	1 cup	1
		22

Total: 65 grams of protein

Recommended Daily Protein Allowance

	AGE yr.	WEIGHT kg. lb.		HEIGHT cm. in.		ENERGY kcal.	PROTEIN gm.
Infants							
	0.0-0.5	6	14	60	24	kg. x 117	kg. x 2.2
	0.5-1.0	9	20	71	28	kg. x 108	kg. x 2.0
Children	1-3	13	28	86	34	1,300	23
	4-6	20	44	110	44	1,800	30 ·
	7-10	30	66	135	54	2,400	36
Males	11-14	44	97	158	63	2,800	44
	15-18	61	134	172	69	3,000	54
	19-22	67	147	172	69	3,000	52
	23-50	70	154	172	69	2,700	56
	51+	70	154	172	69	2,400	56
Females	11-14	44	97	155	62	2,400	44
	15-18	54	119	162	65	2,100	48
	19-22	58	128	162	65	2,100	46
	23-50	58	128	162	65	2,000	46
	51+	58	128	162	65	1,800	46 ·
pregnant						+300	+30
lactating						+500	+20

How Much Protein?

FOOD	AMOUNT	PROTEIN GRAMS	FOOD	AMOUNT	PROTEIN GRAMS
bacon (crisp)	½ ounce	5	salmon, canned, drained	3 ounces	17
beef, cooked	3 ounces	23	shrimp, canned, drained	3 ounces	21
corned beef hash	3 ounces	7	beans (dry, cooked navy, Great Northern, black-eyed peas)	1 cup	13-15
chicken, broiled	3 ounces	20	beans, lima, cooked	1 cup	13
beef heart, braised	3 ounces	27	snap beans, cooked	1 cup	2
chicken pot pie	about 8 ounces before cooking	23	peas, green, cooked	1 cup	9
lamb leg, roasted	3 ounces	23	thin dark green leaves.. cooked spinach, kale, collards, turnip greens	1 cup	4-5
liver beef, fried	3 ounces	22	broccoli, cooked	1 cup	5
pork, roasted	3 ounces	21	Brussels sprouts, cooked	1 cup	7
Braunschweiger, 2 slices, 2-inch diameter, ¼-inch thick	⅔ ounce	3	mushrooms, canned	1 cup	5
frankfurter (one)	2 ounces	7	potatoes, 3 per pound	1 small	3
pork sausage links, 2 links	2 ounces	5	bread, white enriched	1 slice	2
veal, roasted	3 ounces	23	bread, whole-wheat	1 slice	3
clams, raw, meat only	3 ounces	11	bread, light rye, pumpernickel	1 slice	2-3
crabmeat, cooked	3 ounces	15	milk	8 ounces	9
fish, haddock, perch, breaded and fried	3 ounces	17	cheese, cheddar	1 ounce	7
oysters, raw	4 ounces	10	cheese, cottage creamed	¼ cup	8
tuna, canned, drained	3 ounces	24	most fruits	average serving	trace-1
			most vegetables not mentioned	average serving	1-2

Chapter 20

CARBOHYDRATES—THE MILEAGE INGREDIENT

by Eloise R. Trescher, R.D.

Carbohydrates, quite simply, furnish energy. And where would we be without energy? Protein, fat, and alcohol also supply energy, but are less economical sources than carbohydrates. Carbohydrates are the primary and most efficient fuel for muscular exercise in humans.

Composed of carbon, hydrogen, and oxygen, carbohydrates have been aiding man's diet for thousands of years. As early as 8,000 B.C. the cultivation of wild wheats in western Asia freed man of his dependence on hunting and foraging for other foods. Rice has also been a staple in Asia since early times, while in the Americas ancient civilizations grew maize and discovered the value of legumes and potatoes. Honey, another carbohydrate, was used centuries ago but only by royalty and for ceremonial occasions. Today honey is far better spread—from the covering of bread to the spoonfuls on cereal and in tea.

ENERGY FOOD

We get carbohydrates from food. They are widely distributed in the vegetable kingdom and are the least expensive source of energy. The main sources of carbohydrates are starches, sugars, and celluloses. On page 161, is a more detailed guide to help you find carbohydrates when you need them, which is always.

With such a wide variety of foods from which to choose carbohydrates, it is wise to choose those that provide other nutrients. Whole grains are good sources of protein, carbohydrate, thiamin, riboflavin, niacin, iron, and roughage, and when sprouted they supply some ascorbic acid. Bakery products should be made with whole grain or enriched flour. Flours may be labeled "enriched" when prescribed amounts of thiamin, riboflavin, niacin, and iron are added to replace those nutrients removed in the refining process. Dried beans, soybeans, and peas provide the nutrients of whole grains but contribute more protein and iron.

Sugar, honey, jams, jellies, marmalades, preserves, maple and other syrups are a concentrated source of carbohydrates and add variety to the diet. However, they are often referred to as "empty calories," as their contribution of other nutrients is negligible. Remember this when you are giving your child a snack in the afternoon. Instead of a soft drink or a candy bar, why not peel a banana or make a peanut butter and jelly sandwich? The bread, if it is whole grain or enriched, saves the day nutritionally; the jelly is empty but tastes good. Or keep a jar of a mixture of raisins and nuts. Really delicious, you could use 1/3 raisins, 1/3 nuts, 1/3 chocolate bits.

Other sugars such as sorghum and blackstrap molasses furnish carbohydrates, small amounts of calcium, appreciable amounts of iron, and traces of some of the vitamins of the B complex.

Fruits and vegetables provide carbohydrates, minerals, vitamins, water, bulk, and roughage in our diets. Most are relatively low in calories. The juices of fruits and vegetables have all the properties of the foods from which they are made, minus bulk and roughage, but they are a more concentrated source of calories. If you are trying to lose weight, why not an orange rather than a glass of orange juice?

FUEL FOR MUSCLES

Most of the available carbohydrates in our bodies are in the form of glycogen in the skeletal muscles, in the cardiac muscles, and in the smooth muscles. The remaining carbohydrates are present in the manufacturing and distributing systems, in the liver as glycogen, and in the blood and extracellular fluids as glucose. Glycogen in the liver is used as a fuel, has a protective and detoxifying action, and helps regulate protein and fat metabolism. Starvation and disease can deprive the liver of glycogen and so destroy its defenses against many diseases accompanied by toxemias caused by certain bacteria.

An adequate intake of carbohydrate *spares* protein. Less protein is necessary in the diet when generous amounts of carbohydrates are included. When carbohydrates to the liver are limited, fats cannot be completely broken down and ketone bodies are formed, which, if in excess of the amounts that can be oxidized by the peripheral tissues, accumulate in the blood. High levels of ketone bodies cause acidosis and are toxic to tissues such as the brain.

Ketosis can be caused by high-fat–low-carbohydrate diet, by starvation, by glycogen storage disease, by renal glycosuria, by insulin hypoglycemia, in certain conditions where metabolic requirements are increased such as rapid growth, fever, and cold exposure, and by some diseases such as diabetes mellitus.

Amounts of carbohydrates that can be stored in the body are small, but they perform a protective role in some of the most vital organs, such as the heart, the liver, and the central nervous system. Because of the limited amounts of carbohydrates that can be stored in the body it is best to replace them daily, as used. Dr. Robert Goodhart of the New York

Academy of Medicine suggests that a minimum of 100 grams of digestible carbohydrate seems wise in order to avoid ketosis, excessive protein breakdown, involuntary water loss or dehydration, and other problems.

Any of the following combinations would provide about 100 grams of carbohydrates for a day:

I

1 pint milk
1/2 cup lima beans
1/2 cup broccoli
2 slices whole grain or enriched bread
1 orange
1 small apple

II

1 pint milk
1 banana
1/2 cup tomatoes
1/2 cup Brussels sprouts
3 slices whole grain or enriched bread
1/2 grapefruit

III

1 pint milk
1 medium potato
1/2 cup carrots
2 slices whole grain or enriched bread
1/4 cantaloupe
1/2 cup oatmeal

Include carbohydrates in your diet every day. Choose them by the company they keep. Those that provide additional nutrients are your best choice.

Grains rich in carbohydrates and products made from grains are excellent meat extenders, helping you save on that meat bill while offering many nutrients.

Sprouted seeds are another carbohydrate that is becoming more popular, probably because they can be used in so many ways. Try them on sandwiches instead of lettuce, in salads,

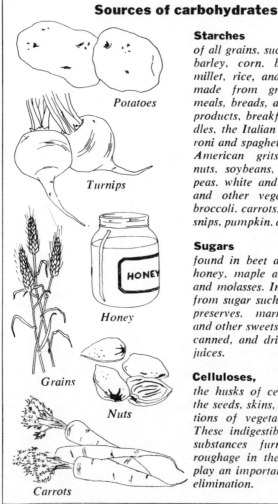

Sources of carbohydrates

Starches

of all grains, such as wheat, rye, barley, corn, buckwheat, flax, millet, rice, and oats. In foods made from grains as flours, meals, breads, and other bakery products, breakfast cereals, noodles, the Italian pastas as macaroni and spaghetti, and the more American grits and hominy. nuts, soybeans, dry beans and peas. white and sweet potatoes, and other vegetables such as broccoli. carrots, kale, okra, parsnips, pumpkin. and turnips.

Sugars

found in beet and cane sugars, honey, maple and corn syrups, and molasses. In products made from sugar such as jams, jellies, preserves. marmalades, candy and other sweets. In fruits, fresh, canned, and dried; and in fruit juices.

Celluloses,

the husks of cereal grains, and the seeds. skins, and fibrous portions of vegetables and fruits. These indigestible and complex substances furnish bulk and roughage in the diet, and they play an important part in aiding elimination.

Potatoes

Turnips

Honey

Grains

Nuts

Carrots

omelettes, homemade bread, and use them when making Chinese dishes. Many seeds may be sprouted, but those that produce the most delicious sprouts are from mung beans, wheat, and alfalfa.

Miki Bond, a Maryland expert who sprouts just about everything, suggests the following method for sprouting seeds; Always pick over seeds carefully, wash them well, then cover with lukewarm water and allow them to soak overnight. Drain and rinse thoroughly. Yield: 1/2 cup seeds swell to 1 1/2 cups after soaking and turn into about 1 quart of sprouts. Place 2 to 3 tablespoons soaked seeds in a quart jar. Cover the top with cheesecloth. Wrap the jar in aluminium foil and place it on its side somewhere warm and dark. Two to three times a day put lukewarm water in the jar, swirl it around, and pour off excess water. Seeds should be moist but not wet. Sprouts develop in 3 to 5 days. When the first young leaves appear, place in direct sunlight for the development of chlorophyll. Wait 8 hours after last rinsing before refrigerating in a closed container.

Chapter 21

WATER—THE ESSENTIAL ELEMENT

by Eloise R. Trescher, R.D.

Only oxygen takes priority over water in maintaining life. Water is vital for all living matter. It is the most essential of all nutrients. This is proved by what it does—its many roles.

WATER WORKS

Water provides the environment in which the body cells live, and plays an active part in forming the building blocks of cells. It also controls the structure and form of the body. It acts as a solvent for all other nutrients and carries them to all parts of the body. Water transports waste products from the body via urine, lungs, the skin, and the feces. It acts as a lubricant in saliva to prevent dryness of mouth and to moisten food, which permits ease of swallowing. Water also helps control body temperature.

Water accounts for one-half to three-fourths of your body weight. It is part of every body cell, muscle, adipose and connective tissue, blood and bone. We can exist for long periods on a diet deficient in other nutrients—protein, fat, carbohydrate, minerals, and vitamins—but we can survive only a few days if deprived of water. Sensations of thirst usually act as a guide to adequate intake of water, infants and sick persons excepted.

Wide variations in water occur because of certain conditions such as excessive sweating, extreme heat, losses from vomiting and diarrhea, high temperatures, retention or excretion due to certain diseases, changes in food mixture, and increases or decreases in certain minerals, such as sodium and potassium, in concert with other minerals.

The mechanisms that control water balance in healthy bodies are exquisitely sensitive and there is little variation between water intake and water output. The healthy kidneys are complex organs which help maintain water balance. They can quickly excrete excess water, and in water deprivation, act to conserve it. In the latter capacity the urine becomes more and more concentrated. There is a constant need for water to rid the body of waste products.

When the body is deprived of water, dehydration quickly occurs as there is a steady loss of water through the lungs and skin by expiration and evaporation. This is called Insensible Water Loss. Body size, the amount of physical activity, and the ambient temperature and humidity influence this water loss. Persons who work hard in high temperatures, such as laborers, soldiers, athletes, and miners, experience excessive water loss. For these individuals there is an increased need for water and sometimes for salt, as there is an excessive loss of this important element in perspiration.

Heat cramps, heat exhaustion, fainting, and heat stroke can result from salt and water imbalance. Heat cramps in skeletal muscles often occur after excessive sweating and drinking large quantities of water. They can be prevented by using small amounts of ordinary table salt in drinking water. All of the above disorders are preventable in healthy individuals if free access to water is provided. Only in profuse sweating is increased intake of salt necessary.

The human adult body contains 30 to 50 liters of water. (A liter is 1.057 quarts.) Total body water as a percentage of body weight is higher in infants, children, and lean adults than in obese individuals. In health, intake and output of water balance closely. If you weigh nude on arising, after voiding, your body weight rarely varies as much as 2 percent and usually less than 1 percent. Water need for the healthy adult is about 1.5 to 2.5 liters a day. Solid and semi-solid foods provide 1,200 to 1,500 milliliters. Beverages account for 1,000 to 1,500 milliliters, and water of oxidation supplies about 300 milliliters from the body's metabolic processes. Water of oxidation may come from several sources:

- 100 grams of protein produce 41.3 grams of water
- 100 grams of starch produce 55.1 grams of water
- 100 grams of fat produce 107.1 grams of water
- 100 grams of alcohol produce 117.4 grams of water

If no food or drink is taken, protein, fat, and glycogen stored in the body tissues are used to supply important amounts of water. It is common knowledge that the camel's hump, made up largely of fat, is a potential source of water.

It is easy to see that many factors influence water balance—many many more than there is space for in this limited discussion. As the Food and Nutrition Board of the National Research Council so succinctly summarized it, "Special attention must be given to the water needs of infants on high protein formulas; of comatose patients; of those with fever, polyuria, vomiting, or diarrhea; of those who are taking diuretics or consuming high-protein diets; and of all persons in hot environments." It should be understood that in most of these circumstances the patient would be under the care of a physician who would determine the required procedure based on the individual's condition.

For the healthy adult, 6 to 8 glasses of fluid a day is a good rule. If you are a slow eater and chew your food thoroughly until it is moistened with sufficient saliva to start the digestive process, liquids may be taken with meals. For those who eat rapidly it is best to take the major part of fluids between meals, as fluids make it easy to swallow food without chewing it sufficiently.

Whether the fluids are hot, cold, or lukewarm, plain or

flavored, is a matter of personal preference and individual physiological response. If you are overweight, choose water. It is free. Tea, coffee, or low-calorie liquids such as artificially sweetened lemonade or limeade might be included in the total daily amount of liquids. If you are on the slender side, choose fruit juices and milk, as they add nutrients as well as fluids.

Percentage of water in a selected list of foods	
Food	Percent of Water
Bacon, *broiled or fried*	8
Uncooked oatmeal	8
Dried beans, *uncooked*	11
Wheat flour	12
Bread, *toasted*	20
Bread, *untoasted*	30
Beef, *cooked*	35-60
Lima beans	71
Avocados	74
Potatoes	80
Apples	85
Oranges	85
Cooked oatmeal	86
Artichokes	86
Milk	87
Orange juice	88
Carrots	90
Watermelon	93
Sugar, *white*	trace
Sugar, *brown*	2
Oils	0

Water is lost from the body each day as follows.

1500 ml. *as urine*
500 ml. *through the skin at average temperature and humidity*
350 ml. *through the expired air at average temp. and humidity*
150 ml. *in feces*
2500 ml.

The person who is constipated may find drinking 2 glasses of water (12 to 16 ounces) on arising helpful. The water should be swallowed rapidly. This activates a quiet gastrointestinal tract and promotes peristaltic waves which propel the fecal mass along the intestinal tract.

For health, water is vital. Yet we often take water for granted. It's hard to believe but true that wars were once waged over water as wars are now waged over oil. A healthy person can live only seven to ten days without it. Don't ever take the value of water for granted; do take it in, regularly every day.

Chapter 22

THE POWER OF POTASSIUM

by Eloise R. Trescher, R.D.

Who would ever expect potassium to turn up on a clambake? Well, if you're a real clambake aficionado, you layer seaweed, a source of potassium, in your cooking pit on the beach. And the Chinese eat their seaweed fried. Potassium is one of the many mineral elements essential to life and responsible for the normal functioning of certain body processes. The chemical symbol for potassium is K. Potassium is concerned with vital biological reactions such as the release and transfer of energy and in protein and glycogen synthesis. It plays a part in transmitting nerve impulses and with magnesium it acts as a muscle relaxant. Potassium is also important in maintaining osmotic pressure and acid-base balance.

The human body is made up of living cells. Potassium contributes an important role in controlling the body's intracellular fluid, while sodium plays a major role in controlling the extracellular fluid. The kidneys tend to excrete potassium along with sodium and water. Therefore, if one is on a low-salt diet, the doctor may wish to increase potassium, especially if one has taken diuretics for a long time. It is generally agreed that potassium supplementation is best accomplished by diet, although in extreme deficiency, medication may be indicated.

Potassium deficiency can result from loss caused by recurrent vomiting, by persistent diarrhea, diabetic acidosis, the use of some diuretic and other drugs, purgatives, and by protein-calorie malnutrition.

Some of the clinical signs of potassium deficiency are extreme muscular weakness, anorexia, lethargy, distention of the intestine, myocardial degenerative changes, and edema of the lungs. The reader should beware of self-diagnosis as all of these symptoms singly and/or collectively are symptoms of many other disorders.

Potassium deficiency usually is associated with other deficiencies of water, calcium, chloride, protein, etc. Potassium intake and output balance well in the *healthy* adult who ingests a nutritionally adequate diet. A deficiency in health rarely occurs as potassium is widely distributed in foods. The Food & Nutrition Board of the National Research Council, 1974, suggests that the healthy adult needs about 2.5 grams of potassium each day. "As with sodium, efficient homeostatic mechanisms allow for a wide range of intake."

In the treatment of some types of heart disease by certain medications, potassium levels in the body may be altered. Other conditions that may need sodium restrictions and potassium supplementation are hypertension, toxemias of pregnancy, edema, certain diseases of the kidneys and liver, and premenstrual tension. Persons taking adrenal cortical steroids may need potassium supplementation.

The amounts of potassium and sodium in foods vary. Fish, meats, poultry, vegetables (including potatoes), fruits, and fruit juices are all good sources of potassium. However, you will see from the table, which shows both sodium and potassium contents of foods, few rules can be made that are foolproof.

These values are compiled from Agriculture Handbook No. 8 on *Composition of Foods, Raw, Processed, Prepared,* U.S. Department of Agriculture, 1963.

Sodium and Potassium in 100 grams or 3 1/3 ounces of selected foods

Food	mg. sodium	mg. potassium
Apples, *raw*	1	110
Apple juice	1	101
Applesauce	2	70
Apricots, *raw*	1	281
Apricots, *canned, water-packed*	1	246
Apricots, *canned, juice-packed*	1	362
Apricots, *canned, syrup-packed*	1	235
Apricot nectar	trace	151
Asparagus, *fresh cooked, boiled, drained*	1	183
Asparagus, *canned, regular pack*	236	166
Asparagus, *low sodium pack*	4	140
Asparagus, *frozen*	1	230
Avocado, *raw*	4	604
Bananas	1	370
Lima beans, *fresh, cooked, boiled, drained*	1	422
Lima beans, *frozen, cooked, boiled, drained*	101	426
Snap beans, *fresh, cooked, boiled, drained*	4	151
Snap beans, *canned, regular pack*	236	95
Snap beans, *low sodium pack*	2	95
Beets, *fresh, cooked, boiled, drained*	43	208
Beets, *canned, regular pack*	236	167
Blackberries, *fresh*	1	170
Blueberries, *fresh*	1	81
Brazil nuts	1	715
Broccoli, *fresh, cooked, boiled, drained*	10	267
Broccoli, *frozen, cooked, chopped, boiled, drained*	15	212
Broccoli spears, *frozen, cooked, boiled, drained*	12	220
Cabbage	20	233
Cabbage, *cooked, boiled, drained*	14	155
Celery, *raw*	126	341
Cherries, *fresh, raw*	2	191
Coffee, *instant liquid beverage*	1	36
Cranberry juice	1	10
Cucumbers, *raw*	6	160
Eggs (chicken) *fresh, uncooked*	122	129
Halibut, *cooked, broiled*	134	525
Lettuce	9	264
Lime juice	1	104
Limeade, *frozen, diluted with 4⅓ parts water*	trace	13

Food	mg. sodium	mg. potassium
Milk, cow's, *whole*	50	144
Milk, goat's	34	180
Milk, human	16	51
Milk, reindeer	157	159
Oranges, *raw, peeled, or juiced*	1	200
Papayas, *raw*	3	234
Peaches, *raw*	1	202
Peanuts, *roasted without salt*	5	701
Peanut butters	605	650
Potatoes, white, *baked in skin, no added salt*	4	503
Pumpkin, *canned without salt*	2	240
Raisins, *uncooked*	27	763
Sauerkraut, *canned*	747	140
Prunes, *dried, uncooked*	11	940
Prunes, *cooked, fruit and liquid*	4	329
Prunes, *dried, uncooked, softened*	8	694
Prunes, *dried, softened, cooked with sugar*	4	327
Prune juice, *canned or bottled*	2	235
Grape juice, *canned or bottled*	2	116
Grape juice, *frozen concentrate diluted with 3 parts water by volume*	1	34
Guavas, *fresh, raw*	4	289
Grapefruit, *raw*	1	135
Grapefruit juice	1	162
Cantaloupe and other varieties	12	251
Watermelon	1	100

It is important to remember that potassium is soluble in water, so foods should be cooked in as little water as possible. Steaming is an excellent method of preparing most vegetables. When there is excess liquid save it for the pot-au-feu. In this way, not only potassium but other water soluble nutrients will be salvaged, too, and the food value of your soups enhanced.

Chapter 23

CALCIUM—THE BACKBONE OF MINERALS

Calcium to many is that glass of milk your mother told you to drink to build better bones. But calcium is much more than a glass of milk—although milk, in all forms, is still the best source of this important mineral.

Everyone should learn more about calcium, as calcium really cares about you from bones to blood. There are more than 100 known elements, and of these calcium (Ca) is present in the largest amounts in the adult human body—2 to 3 pounds, or about 900 to 1,200 grams. Approximately 99 percent of this is in the bone structure and provides the hard part of your bones and teeth. The 1 percent of calcium outside your skeletal structure is in the soft tissues and extracellular fluids.

Contrary to common belief, bone is not fixed, even in adult life. There is a constant altering of its structure by two different kinds of cells. The osteoblasts deposit fresh calcium salts where they are needed, while the osteoclasts erode excess calcium deposits. As hard as bone seems, it is being formed and reabsorbed continuously in your body. About 700 milligrams of calcium enter and leave the bones of the healthy adult every day.

The level of calcium in the blood is maintained with amazing precision at about 9 to 11 milligrams per 100 milliliters in each adult. This relatively small amount performs an immensely important role. It is necessary for the coagulation of the blood (blood clotting), muscle contractility and relaxation, nerve impulse transmission, myocardial (muscular tissue of the heart) function, the integrity of intracellular cement substances and various membranes, and the activation of several enzymes. Calcium, indeed, is both a body builder and a body regulator.

Seventy to eighty percent of the calcium ingested is excreted in the feces, and smaller amounts in urine and sweat. That excreted in the urine varies widely, but research indicates that the amount is fairly constant for each individual.

Our bodies must absorb calcium to have this mineral work for us, and the absorption of calcium is augmented by vitamin D. In areas where there is abundant sunlight there is no need for vitamin D supplementation. In urban areas where pollution may partially obliterate sunlight or where the inhabitants are infrequently exposed to sunlight, vitamin D supplementation may be needed. Remember that vitamin D in excess of need is *toxic* and should be taken *only* when prescribed by your doctor. An adequate intake of lactose (milk is the only source), a low pH (hydrogen ion concentration, which indicates the degree of acidity or alkalinity) of the intestinal contents, the calcium to phosphorus ratio of 1:1, and the need for calcium favor the absorption of calcium.

The level of calcium in the blood of healthy adults is always in balance throughout life. If an adequate amount is not ingested over a long period of time, the level of blood calcium is maintained at the expense of bone. Osteoporosis can occur at any age, but it is most common in postmenopausal women. Its symptoms are a shortening or shrinking of stature often accompanied by low backache and increased incidence of bone fractures.

Many reasons for this phenomenon have been postulated in addition to decreased calcium intake resulting in bone loss. Some of them are: poor absorption, poor utilization, loss of estrogens, and immobility. **Each** plays a part. Older people are less able to absorb calcium than the young. Infirmities may prevent them from engaging in normal activities. Increased calcium intake late in life may not prevent osteoporosis, but it is thought that calcium supplements and increased daily physical activity within the individual's capacity may induce calcium retention and relieve symptoms.

Each person in your family needs calcium throughout life—from infants, children, adolescents, parents, and grandparents to pregnant and lactating women. The table below shows how much calcium should be included in your daily diet.

Age (years)		Calcium milligrams
Infants	0.0-0.5	360
	0.5-1.0	540
Children	1-3	800
	4-6	800
	7-10	800
Males	11-14	1200
	15-18	1200
	19-22	800
	23-50	800
	51+	800
Females	11-14	1200
	15-18	1200
	19-22	800
	23-50	800
	51+	800
Pregnant		1200
Lactating		1200

This table is from the Food and Nutrition Board, National Academy of Sciences, National Research Council, Revised 1974

Authorities vary as to exactly how much calcium an individual needs. For example, the Food and Agricultural Organization of the World Health Organization (FAO/ WHO), suggests that "400 to 500 milligrams per day" of calcium seems "a practical allowance" for adults, as in countries where these amounts are usual, little evidence of calcium deficiency exists. The committee adds, "The usefulness of exceeding this has not been proved. In a number of countries the average intake is considerably higher, in some cases as high as 1500 mg. a day. There is no evidence that such a high intake is undesirable, but neither is there any indication that raising calcium above 1 gram will serve any useful purpose."

The Food and Nutrition Board states, "Studies have shown that men adapt, with time, to lower calcium intakes and maintain calcium balance on intakes as low as 200 to 400 mg. a day, and further, that a higher proportion of calcium is utilized when intake is low than when it is liberal. However, most of the national groups cited as being in equilibrium on such low-calcium intakes either live in tropical or semitropical areas with abundant sunlight or may well have unrecognized sources of calcium in the diet (FAO/WHO 1962). It is therefore unwise to recommend such low calcium intakes."

If foods were listed in the order of their calcium content, milk in its various forms would lead the list, followed by dark green leafy vegetables. Below you will find a list from the U.S. Department of Agriculture Home & Garden Bulletin No. 72 for your kitchen memory board, telling the amount in milligrams of calcium found in a wide variety of food.

It is easy for you to see that milk is our best source of calcium. Include at least 2 glasses in your adult diet each day, either as a beverage, on cereal, in homemade breads, in casseroles, in soups, or in milk desserts. By choosing the remainder of your diet from a wide variety of foods from the four groups you can meet all your nutrient needs.

Guide to calcium content in food

Food	Amount	Calcium Milligrams
Milk (whole)	1 cup (8 oz.)	288
Buttermilk	1 cup (8 oz.)	296

Guide to calcium content in food

Food	Amount	Calcium Milligrams
Milk (skim)	1 cup (8 oz.)	296
Half-and-half	1 cup	261
Light cream	1 cup	203
Heavy cream	1 cup	179
Cheese		
blue or Roquefort	1 ounce	89
Camembert	1⅓ ounce (1 wedge)	40
Cheddar	1 ounce	213
cottage	2 ounces	54
cream	1 ounce	18
Limburger	1 ounce	167
Swiss	1 ounce	262
processed	1 ounce	198
Broccoli, chopped and cooked	1 cup	136
Collards, cooked	1 cup	289
Dandelion greens, cooked	1 cup	252
Turnip greens, cooked	1 cup	252
Spinach, cooked	1 cup	212
Mustard greens, cooked	1 cup	193
Kale, cooked	1 cup	147
Endive, escarole, raw	1 ounce	23
Asparagus, cooked	1 cup	30
Cabbage, cooked in small amount of water	1 cup	64
Cabbage, raw and shredded	1 cup	23
Carrots, cooked, diced	1 cup	48
Celery, raw, diced	1 cup	39
Clams, raw, meat only	3 ounces	59
Oysters, raw, meat only	½ cup	113
Salmon, pink, canned	3 ounces	*167
Sardines, canned	3 ounces	372
Shrimp, cooked	3 ounces	98
Crab meat, canned	3 ounces	38
Beef, lamb, pork, poultry	3 ounces	7 to 10
Molasses (cane) light, first extraction	1 tablespoon	33
blackstrap, third extraction	1 tablespoon	137
Honey, strained	1 tablespoon	17
Sugar, granulated	—	0
Beans		
navy great	1 cup (cooked)	90
kidney	1 cup (cooked)	70
lima	1 cup (cooked)	80
snap	1 cup (cooked)	63
Peanuts	10 jumbo	13
Peanut butter	2 level tablespoons	18
Almonds	10	23
Brazil nuts	8 medium	25
Bread, whole-wheat	1 1-ounce slice	32
Bread, white enriched	1 1-ounce slice	25
Pumpernickel	1 1-ounce slice	27

Guide to calcium content in food

Food	Amount	Calcium Milligrams
Egg yolk	1 large	24
Strawberries	1 cup	31
Orange	1 large	81
Orange	1 medium	65
Orange	1 small	52
Orange juice	1 cup	25
Cantaloupe	½ (5-inch dia.)	38
Apples	1 (3 per pound)	10
Waffle, made with enriched flour	1-2½ ounces (4-inch dia.)	85
Waffle, made from mix, enriched, egg and milk added	as above	179
Wheat, shredded	1 biscuit	11
Spaghetti, cooked	1 cup	32
Spaghetti, home recipe with meatballs and sauce	1 cup	124
Spaghetti, canned	1 cup	53

If bones are discarded, calcium value will be greatly reduced

Here are three delicious recipes with calcium in mind:

Mrs. Joe Hume Gardner's Scalloped Cabbage with Nutmeg Sauce

Ingredients

1 small head cabbage, coarsely shredded
2 tablespoons butter or margarine
2 tablespoons flour
1½ cups milk
½ teaspoon salt
Few grains pepper
¼ teaspoon nutmeg
6 tablespoons grated Parmesan cheese
1 tablespoon lemon juice

Method

Boil or steam cabbage until tender, but still crisp. Melt butter in saucepan. Stir in flour.

Remove from heat and gradually blend in milk, stirring till smooth. Add salt, pepper, and nutmeg, stirring constantly until thickened. Add 4 tablespoons cheese and stir until melted. Remove from heat and stir in lemon juice.

Place cabbage in greased baking dish. Pour over sauce. Top with remaining cheese and a light sprinkle of nutmeg. Bake in hot (450°) oven 6–8 minutes, until top is golden brown. Serves 6.

Mrs. William W. Magruder's Broccoli Mold

Ingredients
2 10-ounce packages frozen chopped broccoli
2 tablespoons unflavored gelatin
1 10½-ounce can consommé
2 tablespoons lemon juice
1 teaspoon red hot sauce
½ teaspoon salt
½ cup mayonnaise
3 hard-cooked eggs, chopped
½ cup celery, chopped (optional)
½ cup slivered almonds

Method
Cook broccoli according to package directions. Soak gelatin in ½ cup consommé for 5 minutes. Heat remaining consommé. Add to gelatin mixture. Stir to dissolve.

Drain broccoli. Combine remaining ingredients. Add consommé-gelatin mixture.

Pour into mold and chill until firm. Unmold onto platter of salad greens. May be garnished with black olives, cocktail tomatoes, or whatever is handy. Serves 8 to 10.

Mrs. John M. Young's Buttermilk Dressing

Ingredients
2 cups mayonnaise
1¼ cups buttermilk
½ teaspoon garlic salt
1 teaspoon Worcestershire sauce
Dash of Tabasco
4 ounces blue cheese

Method
Mix all ingredients in blender, putting in cheese last.

(These three recipes are taken from the 1977 *Stratford Hall Cookbook*.)

Chapter 24

WHOLE GRAINS AND OTHER NATURAL FIBERS

by Eloise R. Trescher, R.D.

> Said a lean, wiry lipid imbiber
> Of no diet am I a subscriber
> And you never would guess
> That I eat to excess
> For the secret, my friends, is the fiber.
>
> (From an article by Dr. David Kritchevsky, The Wistar Institute of Anatomy and Biology, Philadelphia, Pennsylvania.)

The implication of the above limerick is yet to be proven, but research in this country and in England has turned up convincing evidence to establish its credibility.

What is dietary fiber? It is that part of plants, the whole grains, vegetables, nuts, fruits, and legumes that are not digested by the secretions of the human gastrointestinal tract. It is made up of a complex of carbohydrates of which the layman rarely hears—celluloses, hemicelluloses, mucilages, pentosans, gums, pectins, and non-carbohydrate lignin.

Recently research has revived interest in dietary fiber. But as early as 1920, Dr. J. H. Kellogg, Medical Director of the Battle Creek Sanatorium, advised an "Antitoxic Diet." He recommended the daily use of fruits, vegetables, nuts, legumes, and whole grain cereals, especially coarse oatmeals and wheat bran in our diets.

Dr. Kellogg wrote, "Modern medical research has clearly incriminated the colon as the source of more disease and physical suffering than any other organ of the body. The artificial conditions of life, sedentary habits, concentrated foodstuffs, false modesty, ignorance, and neglect of bodily needs have provided a crippled state of the colon as an almost universal condition among civilized men and women. One of the many functions of the colon or large intestine is to carry food residue to the rectum."

In 1974, fifty-four years later, Dr. B. H. Ershoff wrote in the *Journal of Applied Nutrition* the following possible benefits of dietary fiber:

1. As an anti-hypercholesterolemic and anti-atherosclerotic agent (prevention of an elevated cholesterol and hardening of the arteries).

2. As a promoter of normal bowel function.

3. As an antitoxic agent.

The multimillion dollar annual sales of laxatives and cathartics substantiate their claims. Present studies indicate that diets low in fiber might be implicated in certain types of heart disease, elevated cholesterol, cancer of the colon, and other diseases of the colon such as diverticulosis.

The ways in which dietary fiber works are complex. Different kinds of fiber play different roles. The chief roles of dietary fibers are to:

1. Increase the bulk of the diet. This may result in greater excretion of bile salts and fats.

2. Permit greater water-binding capacity of the intestinal contents.

3. Promote a favorable milieu for intestinal bacterial flora.

4. Produce larger and softer stools.

5. Decrease the transit time of the fecal mass. Carcinogenic substances would have shorter contact time with the intestinal mucosa and therefore less chance of promoting the development of cancer.

Persons whose diets are composed of highly refined foods and foods low in fiber content (meat, fish, poultry, eggs, cheese) are often constipated and take muciloids in water to provide intestinal bulk. A happier solution to the problem is to eat foods high in fiber content—a salad of fresh fruit or greens; 100 percent whole grain breads, crackers, or cereals, especially those rich in bran; some dried figs or prunes; a dish of Scotch oatmeal at breakfast. Any of these, singly or in combination, provide pleasant ways of including dietary fiber, and help promote satisfactory bowel movements.

Little is known about the specific properties of different fibers. The U.S. Department of Agriculture Handbook No. 8, 1963, our most recent comprehensive source of information on the composition of foods, lists only crude fiber, or C.F. Crude fiber is the insoluble material left after severe acid-base hydrolysis. C.F. values must be used because those for dietary fibers are presently unavailable.

The amounts of C.F. in foods vary widely. Whole grains contain large quantities, but as you see in the lists, much is removed in milling. The C.F. of some selected foods may serve as a guide in helping you to increase the fiber content of your family meals. Consult it. Use it.

Years of research will be necessary before the true role of fibers will be delineated. In the interim choose your family meals from a wide variety of foods. Variety adds interest and insures that both the discovered and yet-to-be-discovered nutrients are included.

Foods	Approximate amounts of crude fiber (percent)
Wheat bran	7.8
Wheat germ	2.5
Whole wheat bread	1.6
Pumpernickel	1.1
White bread	.2
Rice bran	11.5
Brown rice, cooked	.3
Polished rice, cooked	.1
Green peas, cooked	2.2
Split peas without seed coat, cooked	4.4
Lentils with seed coat, cooked	1.2
Soy beans, cooked	1.4
Beans, cooked	
Green, snap	1.
Ford Hook limas	1.6
Baby limas	1.9
Navy, marrow fat	1.5
Mung beans, sprouted	.7
Peanuts, roasted	2.4
Peanut butter	1.8
Almonds	2.6
Popcorn, popped	2.2
Walnuts, English	2.1
Brazil nuts	3.1
Walnuts, black	1.7
Prunes, dried, uncooked	2.2
Prunes, "softenized," uncooked	1.6
Dates, dried	2.3
Figs, dried, uncooked	5.6
Figs, fresh, raw	1.2
Figs, cooked	.7
Orange, peeled fruit	.5
Orange juice	.1
Apples, not pared	1.
Apples, pared	.6
Apricots, dried, uncooked	3.8
Apricots, cooked	.9
Kumquats, fresh, raw	3.7
Blueberries, fresh, raw	1.5
Strawberries, fresh, raw	1.3
Blackberries, fresh, raw	4.1
Asparagus, cooked	.7
Avocado, raw	1.5
Beets, cooked	.8
Tomatoes, raw	.5

Foods	Approximate amounts of crude fiber (percent)
Spinach, cooked	.7
Corn, fresh, cooked	.7
Lettuce	.5
Carrots	1.
Cauliflower	1.
Broccoli	1.5
Cabbage	.8
Meat, fish, poultry, eggs, cheese	0

Here are three recipes to try and enjoy. Each provides a good source of fiber and is delicious.

Bran Muffins

Ingredients
2 cups graham flour
1½ cups bran
2 tablespoons sugar
¼ teaspoon salt
1¼ teaspoons soda
2 cups sour milk
1 beaten egg
½ cup blackstrap molasses
2 tablespoons melted butter
½ cup raisins
½ cup nutmeats

Method
Combine and stir well the graham flour, bran, sugar, salt, and soda. Beat together the milk, egg, molasses, butter. Combine the dry and liquid ingredients with a few swift strokes. Fold in raisins and nutmeats. Bake the muffins in a moderate (350°) oven for about 25 minutes. Makes about twenty-two 2-inch muffins. Adapted from *The Joy of Cooking*.

Two of my younger friends—Tommy, nineteen, and Beth, seventeen—suggested the next two recipes.

Wheat-Soy Waffles

Ingredients
1 cup whole wheat flour
1 teaspoon salt
¼ cup soy flour
2 teaspoons baking powder
2 eggs, separated
1½ cups milk
3 tablespoons melted butter or oil
2 tablespoons honey

Method
Stir dry ingredients together. Beat egg yolks, add milk, butter, and honey and blend well. Stir into dry ingredients. Beat the egg whites until stiff and fold them into the batter. Bake on hot, oiled waffle iron. Makes about 10 waffles. You can add ½ cup of chopped nuts folded in with the egg whites. From *Diet for a Small Planet* by Frances Moore Lappe.

Lacy Oatmeal Cookies

Ingredients
½ pound butter, melted
2¼ cups light brown sugar
2¼ cups regular oatmeal (not instant)
1 teaspoon vanilla
1 egg slightly beaten

Method
Mix together the melted butter, sugar, oatmeal, vanilla, and egg. Drop by the teaspoonful on an ungreased cookie sheet, allowing for 3-inch spread. Bake in 350° oven until

brown, 5–7 minutes. Cool the cookies. Makes 5 dozen. Contributed by Mrs. Richard Randall to the Walters Art Gallery cookbook, *Private Collections.*

Rice Bread

Ingredients
2 tablespoons dry yeast
1½ cups lukewarm water
¼ cup honey
2 cups cooked, moist rice
2 tablespoons corn or rice oil
2 teaspoons salt
½ cup rice bran
5 cups unbleached flour

Method
Preheat oven to 375°. In a large bowl, mix yeast, water, and honey until dissolved and frothy. Thoroughly blend in rice, oil, salt and rice bran. Add enough flour to form a soft dough. Knead dough on floured board at least 15 minutes until smooth and elastic. Form into ball, place in greased bowl, cover with damp tea towel and set in warm place to rise 1½ hours or until double in size. Punch down, let rise again 40 minutes or until doubled and return to floured board. Knead and shape into 2 loaves, place in 2 greased bread pans and let rise until again double in size. Bake for 10 minutes, lower heat to 325°, and continue baking 35 minutes. Remove from oven; let stand 5 minutes; remove from pans and cool on rack. Makes 2 loaves. From *Ricecraft* (Yerba Buena Press) by Margaret Gin.

Chapter 25

NUTRITION LABELING—PROOF OF THE PUDDING

by Eloise R. Trescher, R.D.

Nutrition labeling, a project begun in 1973 by the Food and Drug Administration (FDA), is alive and well. It is designed to provide practical and reliable nutrition information for consumers, enabling us to make intelligent food choices, compare food products, and feel assured of a good selection. It is expected to improve the nutritive quality of foods and increase consumer confidence in the food industry.

Reading labels is an appetizer, a mini-course in nutrition, arousing our interest to learn more. At present, nutrition labeling is voluntary. It is mandatory only when a nutrient is added to a food to replace nutrients lost during processing, for fortification, *or* when an advertising claim is made for the nutritional value of a food, such as "high in," "rich in," "excellent," "good," "packed," or "loaded." Additional rulings of the FDA have been well-summarized by the National Dairy Council:

"A claim cannot be made that a particular food is a significant source of a nutrient per serving unless that nutrient exists in the food in an amount equal to or in excess of 10 percent of the U.S. RDA (United States Recommended Daily Dietary Allowance) for that nutrient per serving. Labeling claims may not suggest or imply the following:

1. That a food is beneficial in the prevention, cure, mitigation, or treatment of a disorder;

2. That a balanced diet of conventional foods contributes an insufficient amount of nutrients;

3. That a suboptimal nutrient profile of a food, due to soil composition in which the food was grown, contributes to an inadequate daily dietary intake;

4. That various food processing and handling techniques result in a deficient daily diet;

5. That the food has dietary attributes when those properties are of no consequence in human nutrition;

6. That natural vitamins in food are superior to added vitamins."

As indicated on the label (see end of chapter) nutrition information includes serving size, number of servings per container, calories, and the amount of protein, fat, and carbohydrate in grams (a gram is about one-thirtieth of an ounce). The listing of eight nutrients is mandatory, *even* if only two nutrients are removed in processing, then added. They must be listed in this order:

> Protein
> Vitamin A
> Vitamin C
> Thiamin
> Riboflavin
> Niacin
> Calcium
> Iron

They must also be expressed as a percentage of the U.S. RDA. Other nutrients may be listed, but *must* be listed if added to a food. If a serving of food contains less than 2% of a nutrient of the U.S. RDA this is noted by an asterisk and the statement "Contains less than 2% of the U.S. RDA of these nutrients."

Many people do not know that the "ingredients" part of a label must list every ingredient included in the food product in the order of its concentration. The item, or ingredient, present in the largest amount is listed first, and so on down the line. The labels on this page and on page 192 demonstrate this and show relative proportions of an ingredient at a quick glance. For example, in the bottom label, where vegetable oil follows salt, you can be sure that there is very little vegetable oil in the product.

```
                     ENRICHED
PRECOOKED RICE, SUGAR,
SALT, GARLIC POWDER,
DRIED RED AND GREEN BELL
PEPPERS WITH SULFUR DI-
OXIDE ADDED AS A PRESER-
VATIVE, PAPRIKA, DRIED
ONION, HYDROLYZED VEGE-
TABLE PROTEIN (FOR FLA-
VOR), SPICE, CARAMEL
COLOR.              170 G.
```

```
PREPARED FROM: TOMATOES, EN-
RICHED WHEAT FLOUR, SUGAR,
SALT, VEGETABLE OIL, NATURAL
SPICE OILS AND VITAMIN C.
```

In an interview in *U.S. News & World Report,* Dr. Alexander M. Schmidt, former Commissioner of the Food and Drug Administration, outlined the increasing concern of the consumer about drugs, chemicals, the ozone layer, and food. He attributes this concern to the increase in scientific knowledge and the demands of the better-educated consumer for action to avoid hazards that the scientists are discovering.

To answer the question, "Just how safe are the things we eat?" he responded: "Basically our food supply is safer than it has ever been, no question at all. With all the concern over food additives* we tend to overlook the fact that

---

* The FDA does not decide whether food and color additives may be used. This is done by congressional legislation. All the FDA does is try to determine through research which food and color additives are legally safe enough to be used in food.

hazards from additives are very small, infinitesimal really, compared with risks that were in food years ago and that now have been reduced to practically zero.

"There is less microbiological contamination than ever before because manufacturing processes are getting better all the time. As an example, the amount of lead in juices and baby foods has been halved since 1973. Heavy-metal contamination in food is at its all-time low right now and sinking fast."

When asked, "What is the big danger in our food supply today?" Dr. Schmidt said: "Bacterial contamination of food still leads our list of hazards. More than two million people a year in this country get sick from what we commonly call food poisoning, but most cases result from poor handling of food while it is being prepared or stored."

Americans want really sound information on nutrition. The National Nutrition Consortium, Inc., can help. A dependable source, this organization was also founded in 1973 "with the purpose of promoting the health and well-being of the American people." The Consortium is made up of leaders from six major societies and represents more than 50,000 members of various food and science organizations.

The six societies of the Consortium are:

1. The American Dietetic Association, the national professional organization for dietitians.

2. The American Society for Clinical Nutrition, an organization of physicians and scientists engaged in clinical nutrition research.

3. The American Institute of Nutrition, whose membership includes university, government, and industry researchers in nutrition, biochemistry, and physiology.

4. The Institute of Food Technologists, a professional society concerned with techniques for improving the food supply.

5. The Society for Nutrition Education, whose goal is more effective nutrition education.

6. The American Academy of Pediatrics, an association of pediatricians whose primary purpose is insuring the "attainment by all children of the Americas of their full potential for physical, emotional, and social health."

The Consortium's booklet *Nutrition Labeling* contains far more information than its name implies. In concise, easily understood language it explains all that most of us need to know about calories, proteins, carbohydrates, fats, cholesterol, sodium, U.S. RDA's recommended daily dietary allowances, vitamins, and minerals (both those which *must* be listed and those which *may* be listed), how to make the most of label information, plus four appendixes and an index. Rarely is so much useful information presented in so few (134) pages. The booklet can help you assess advertisers' nutrition claims and understand nutrition labeling at a glance.

Nutrition Labeling is $2 postpaid and may be obtained from the National Nutrition Consortium, Inc., P.O. Box 4110, Kankakee, Illinois, 60901. Order it; read it. With a sound knowledge of nutrition, you can plan well-blanced meals for your family at less cost than you thought possible in these days of skyrocketing food prices.

This booklet concerns itself only with the consumer. The work of the Food and Drug Administration on nutrition labeling, however, also concerns the manufacturers, the regulatory agencies, and educators. The FDA is not only alive and well, but working hard.

NET WT. 10½ OZ. 298 GRAMS
HEAT & SERVE OR USE COLD FOR SALADS
Ingredients:
Cut Green Asparagus, Water, Salt.

NUTRITION INFORMATION
Serving Size . . . . 1 cup
Servings per Container . . . 1¼
(or 3 3½-oz. servings)

Per One-Cup Serving:
Calories 40   Carbohydrate . . 5 gm
Protein . . . 3 gm   Fat . . . . 1 gm

PERCENTAGE OF U.S. RECOMMENDED DAILY ALLOWANCE (U.S. RDA)
Protein 4   Riboflavin . . . 6
Vitamin A . . . 15   Niacin 6
Vitamin C . . . 60   Calcium 2
Thiamine 4   Iron 2

Chapter 26

HOW TO PLAN NUTRITIONALLY SOUND VEGETARIAN MEALS

by Eloise R. Trescher, R.D.

Several years ago, a popular and now-famous cartoon in *The New Yorker* showed a mother and young daughter sitting at the dinner table. The mother was trying to persuade her daughter to eat and the child was rebellious. Mother says, "It's broccoli, dear." And the daughter answers, "I say it's spinach, and I say the hell with it!" That precocious child just might be eating her words and have an entirely different slant on spinach if she were pictured today. So very many of our young are turning more and more to vegetables and vegetarianism. And in turn teaching their elders about it.

In the past, vegetarianism was practiced largely for religious, cultural, ethnic, or moral reasons. But the recent boom in population and food shortages throughout most of the world have evoked fresh interest in and new converts to vegetarianism. Recently biochemists have done more intensive research on the adequacy of proteins of vegetable origins. Nutritionists when planning diets favor a wide variety in the selection of foods and include some foods of animal origin for their good protein, B vitamins, and mineral content.

The motives that inspire the renewed interest in vegetarianism range from compassion to fanaticism. Many persons object to the killing of animals, birds, and fish for food. Others entertain beliefs based on Eastern philosophies, with which they are only vaguely familiar, or biochemical misinformation, which they really don't understand. And who isn't complaining about rising costs of food, especially meat? Vegetarians aren't.

Regardless of motives, a lacto-ovo vegetarian regime can be nutritious and satisfying and reduce food bills in many instances. It can increase the fiber content of one's diet, and, very importantly, reduce the fat and cholesterol found in typical American diets. It can also help control weight. Most adult vegetarians weigh 10 to 20 pounds less than their meat-eating peers. The variety of foods eaten is expanded and menus are likely to be more interesting.

Vegetarians may be divided into four groups:

1. *Strict vegetarians,* the "Vegans." They eat no food of animal sources: meat, fish, poultry, milk, eggs, or cheese.

2. *Lacto-ovo vegetarians.* These include eggs, milk, and milk products in their diets.

3. *Lacto-vegetarians.* They allow themselves milk and milk products in their diets.

4. *Ovo-vegetarians.* Eggs are included in this diet.

The "Vegans" are the only ones of the above four groups in danger of malnutrition. The effects of strict avoidance of food of animal origin may not be apparent for many years, perhaps twelve to fifteen. Long-term "Vegans" are relatively rare, but they are likely sooner or later to suffer the destruction of certain nerve fibers. This condition is irreversible, caused by a lack of vitamin B_{12}. There is no adequate source of B_{12} in the vegetable kingdom. However, this important vitamin could be taken as medication.

Another hazard of the strict vegetarian diet is calcium deficiency, which doesn't show up until late in life in the form of bone fractures. All *strict* vegetable diets are likely to be low in calcium, and the calcium from medication is not as efficiently utilized as from food. Such calcium deficient diets are especially hazardous for the infant, the growing child and adolescent, and the pregnant or lactating mother. Other possible nutritional deficiencies of the "Vegans" are iron and iodine. There are relatively few food sources of vitamin D. Food sources of vitamin D are cod liver and other fish liver oils. Increasingly, milk is being fortified with vitamin D, but not everywhere. Where there is very little opportunity for exposure to the sun, vitamin D, which is necessary for calcium utilization, may be lacking. Vitamin D may be supplied by medication.

Despite the above seemingly ominous warnings, it is possible to obtain an adequate diet from the vegetable world by supplementing it with vitamin B_{12}. However, this requires a broad knowledge of the dietary properties of foods.

Amino acids, and there are 22 of them, are the building blocks of protein. The word "protein" is of Greek origin, meaning "primary" or "of first importance." Protein is essential for every living organism. If vegetarianism is to be your route, the lacto-ovo vegetarian diet is the wisest, the diet that includes, along with vegetables, eggs, milk, and milk products.

The healthy individual can synthesize within his or her own body 14 amino acids. The other 8 (leucine, lysine, valine, isoleucine, threonine, phenylalanine, methionine, and tryptophan) must be obtained from food. These 8 have been labeled "essential amino acids." All 8 are present in foods of animal origin except gelatin. In foods of vegetable origin, such as cereal grains, nuts, legumes, vegetables, and fruit, one or more of these essential amino acids may be missing. However, by eating certain *combinations* of foods, our amino acid needs may be met. That is, the presence of an amino acid in one food may supply that amino acid in which another food is lacking. One of the more classic examples of this complementing action is found in beans and rice.

Long before researchers discovered the scientific reasons for using these two foods "in combination," people in many parts of the world were eating them and thriving. One can only marvel at the wisdom of these people, much of it learned no doubt from long and bitter experience. Here is a recipe for complementing beans and rice:

Baked Bean and Brown Rice Rarebit

Ingredients
3 onions
4 tablespoons butter
1 #2 can solid pack tomatoes
1 cup cooked brown rice
1 can baked beans
1 pound extra-sharp cheese, grated
Salt and pepper to taste

Method
Chop onions and sauté in butter until golden. Add tomatoes, cooked rice, and beans and heat until just below the boiling point. Add grated cheese and cook over low heat until cheese melts. Season to taste. Serve on toasted Boston brown bread or toasted English muffins. This is better if made ahead of time and reheated. Serves 6 to 10.

Here's a lacto-vegetarian recipe:

Kay Lewis's Vegetable Casserole

Ingredients
1 package frozen Brussels sprouts
1 jar (1½ to 2 cups) canned carrots
1 jar (1½ to 2 cups) small onions
1 can cream of mushroom soup
¼ cup milk
Parmesan cheese, grated

Method

Preheat oven to 350°. Place all ingredients except cheese in a casserole. Sprinkle cheese on top. Bake until cooked, about 25–30 minutes. Serves 6 to 8.

Seventh Day Adventists have long practiced the lacto-ovo vegetarian diet. Its nutritional adequacy is unquestioned, and it is a well-documented fact that the general health of the members of this religious sect is good and their life span is somewhat longer than meat eaters.

Recently a friend of mine spent ten days, her children's spring holiday, cooking lacto-ovo vegetarian meals. The children's ages range from twenty-two to seventeen, and this course of food preparation was suggested by her elder son who happens to attend the agricultural college of Cornell, and is majoring in "Vegetables." She laughed at first, found it a challenge, enjoyed it, and became convinced of its value. It was fun, especially planning the menus with the children, learning with them, and for the first time she found her children cooking with her as a family.

Here are three recipes her family thought delicious and found easy to make. All come from *Diet for a Small Planet* by Frances Moore Lappé.

Spinach Casserole

Ingredients
¾ cup raw brown rice, cooked
½ cup grated Cheddar cheese
2 eggs, beaten
2 tablespoons parsley, chopped
½ teaspoon salt
¼ teaspoon pepper
1 pound fresh spinach, chopped
2 tablespoons wheat germ
1 teaspoon butter, melted

Method

Preheat oven to 350°. Combine the cooked rice and cheese. Combine the eggs, parsley, salt, and pepper. Add the two mixtures together and stir in the raw spinach. Pour into an oiled casserole. Top the spinach with wheat germ mixed with the melted butter. Bake for 35 minutes. Serves 4.

Potato Latkes

Ingredients
2 eggs
½ onion, cubed
1 large potato, cubed
salt and pepper to taste
2 tablespoons whole wheat flour
2 tablespoons chopped parsley
5 tablespoons instant dry milk
oil for frying

Method

Blend eggs, onion, and potato cubes in a blender. Then add and blend salt and pepper, whole wheat flour, parsley, and powdered milk. Using this batter, fry like small pancakes in hot oil. Brown both sides well. Top with applesauce, yoghurt, or soft cheese. Or just eat them plain. Serves 2 to 3, for breakfast, lunch, or supper.

This next recipe is filled with protein. Served with a green salad it is a beautifully balanced nutritious meal. The family that tried these recipes also made additions to this one. They cooked it as written here and also varied it by adding a cup of finely chopped broccoli to the mixture; another time they added a layer of thinly sliced tomatoes. Any way it was done, it was a big success.

Easy Cheese Soufflé

Ingredients
3 cups grated cheese
4–6 slices bread
2 cups milk or 1½ cups milk and ½ cup wine or vermouth
3 eggs, beaten
½ teaspoon salt
½ teaspoon Worcestershire sauce
½ teaspoon dry mustard
½ teaspoon thyme
Pepper to taste

Method
Preheat oven to 350°. Layer the cheese and bread in an oiled baking dish, starting with the bread. Pour over it the milk or milk mixture. Beat with the eggs the remaining ingredients and pour over the bread mixture. Let stand for 30 minutes. Bake one hour in a pan of hot water. In a deep dish it has the appearance of a soufflé; in a shallow dish, it resembles a quiche.

After reading this, you might want to try a delicious and nutritionally adequate lacto-ovo vegetarian diet for a day or two, or even more. This diet offers such variety. So why not explore?

SOME SOUND GUIDELINES FOR VEGETARIANS:

Be sure your calorie needs are met: 2,000 calories for a healthy woman aged twenty-three to fifty whose weight is within normal limits, and 2,700 for a man aged twenty-three to fifty. Choose your diet from a wide variety of whole cereal grains, nuts, soybeans, and other "oil seeds," thin dark green leaves, other vegetables, millets, legumes, and fruits.

Be sure your protein needs are met: 46 grams of protein

each day for a healthy woman age twenty-three to fifty and 56 grams for a man aged twenty-three to fifty. These are the recommended daily dietary allowances from the Food and Nutrition Board of the National Research Council. For example, a typical day's meals might include:

	Grams of Protein
3 glasses of milk	24
4 slices of whole grain bread	8
⅔ cup cooked dried beans, peas, or lentils °	10
2 ounces cheese	14

(The inclusion of milk, milk products, and eggs enhances the quality of the vegetarian diet in all probably deficient areas except iodine. Using iodized salt provides this important trace element.)

° or 1 egg   7

Part Three

WEIGHT CONTROL FOR A HEALTHY BODY

Eating right also means keeping control of your weight. New diets appear every year, but the wisest course is to use common sense and listen to the experts. Here you will find advice from nutritionists and psychologists, plus menus and exclusive recipes from five world-famous spas, and low-calorie entertaining ideas.

Chapter 27

WEIGHT CONTROL—THE BASICS

by Eloise R. Trescher, R.D.

The subject of nutrition is coming into its own. Never before has so much been written on the how, when, where, and what to eat. The public is becoming aware. The word is spreading. But not quite as fast as American waistlines. Weight control is one of our country's main health problems. Obesity should be looked upon as a disease, not a vice.

Controlling your weight is really controlling your destiny. To think thin is more than being fashionable; it's being sensible. As Hippocrates wrote long ago, "Persons who are very fat are apt to die earlier than those who are slender." Times haven't changed.

I once had a patient, a deeply religious woman, who wanted to lose "so I can get down on my knees to pray." Another was an employee of a gas and electric company who couldn't get his rotund self into the manhole containing the machinery he was required to operate. The rewards of losing weight on a nutritionally adequate basic regimen are legion. You improve your entire physical condition, your vitality, your resistance to fatigue as well as your mental alertness. You'll be a much happier person, proud of your own self-image.

Medically speaking, the overweight are asking for trouble. They are much more likely to develop diabetes, high blood pressure, and hardening of the arteries than the slender individual. The overweight are poor surgical risks. Stout women often have menstrual disorders, are less likely to conceive, and have more complications with pregnancies than leaner women. Gout and gallstones are other unwelcome companions to the overweight, as well as shortness of breath, mechanical limitations, varicosities, and joint and back pains. Nowadays no one *really* loves a fat man. Much less himself.

We become overweight when we take in more calories than we need for the energy we put out. Calories measure the energy our bodies receive from various foods. These amounts vary according to their fat, carbohydrate, and protein content. And quite simply we need this energy to live. What we must remember is to balance the energy we eat against the energy we use. Eating nutritionally and exercising moderately is the answer. It is far easier to prevent overweight than to cure it.

Good food habits at any age do not just happen. Left to his own devices, a child may form habits of overeating that may continue through adulthood. Psychological factors often contribute to overweight when the individual's social, occupational, professional, or sexual desires are unfulfilled.

Overweight often develops insidiously in individuals who do not seem to eat excessively. As little as 100 calories a day in excess of one's needs can result in a gain of 10 to 12 pounds a year. Think how you might look in five more years! Try on a skirt or dress you wore when you were twenty-five, considering you were in reasonable shape. If the zipper doesn't meet, you should meet the challenge and start losing weight right now.

Nor do you have to be a Billie Jean King when it comes to exercising off calories. A brisk walk for half an hour will burn an average of 150 calories. Although it's not as invigorating, you'll burn just as many calories if you make beds for half an hour. Perhaps more entertaining would be dancing, but fast— 600 calories an hour. Whatever your activity, it should be on a daily, year-in, year-out basis. Along with using energy and helping to control your weight, physical activity improves circulation of the blood and improves muscle tone. It helps lessen tension and fatigue and gives one a sense of mental alertness and physical well-being.

There is no "Master Diet" that will fit *all* people. A good maxim is "Arrest weight gain." Lives are too variable and people too individualized for anyone to evolve a set of rules—but there are ways:

Decrease calorie intake. If you stop eating an extra 25 calories or so a day, you might stop gaining weight. And if you cut back 100 calories a day less than your needs, you will lose 10 to 12 pounds a year.

Learn to eat slowly and chew thoroughly.

Limit portions of food at meals to one average serving.

Never take second helpings.

Omit or drastically restrict free fats—butter, margarine, mayonnaise, salad oils, cooking fats. Sufficient fat is present in lean meats, fish, poultry, eggs, and cheese to insure adequate use of the fat soluble vitamins, A, D, E, and K.

Omit or drastically restrict free sweets—jelly, jam, honey, syrups, sugar, candy, pies, pastries, and most other desserts.

Restrict or eliminate intake of alcoholic beverages.

Eat a good breakfast and never skip a meal.

Never use food as a reward.

Learn to practice moderation. If you decide to indulge in a high-calorie food, eat it slowly and eat one half or less than you normally would.

Buy a good scale and use it. Weigh once a week and keep a written record of your weight.

Never go grocery shopping when hungry. Before starting off, have a piece of fruit, a glass of skim milk, a cup of bouillon, some raw vegetables. This will probably stop aisle-to-aisle munching.

Keep a food diary (see Chapter 29). Record in detail food and drink for a week. This helps stiffen resistance to dietary temptations. It is also an important aid in that it may reveal unconscious departures.

Few adults know that a reduction of approximately 75–

100 calories per day, after the age of thirty-five, is a must if the healthy individual is permanently to achieve weight control. You must accept the fact that you did not become fat overnight and that you cannot shed those unwanted pounds quickly. The more gradual the change in one's food habits, the more likely the moderation is to become a permanent habit, a new way of life.

If Jack Sprat and his wife had known more about nutrition, another old nursery rhyme might have been deleted from young children's literary diets. One only ate lean, the other only fat. A healthy individual should include food from all four food groups every day (see page 129).

The amount of food needed depends on one's height, age, sex, skeletal structure, and activity. At the present time few doctors are trained to give the specific detailed instructions most persons requiring dietary advice need, nor do they have the time. But the doctor does know his patient's physical condition and any weight alteration should not be attempted or considered except by his approval.

A doctor knows resources and should be able to put his patient in the hands of a qualified diet therapist or nutritionist who will plan with the patient the diet best suited to his needs, provide written instructions, detailed advice, and periodic checkups. Of greatest importance is moral support and encouragement from the therapist and physician. Each will emphasize the importance of a nutritionally sound "Foundation Diet." And the patient must understand that *including* the right kind of food in the correct quantities is as important, or more so, to his well being than *excluding* certain foods.

Never forget that the best diet to reduce weight must restrict calories without restricting essential nutrients, as well as provide a certain amount of gastronomic satisfaction. The person supplied with a diet tailored to his individual needs and who has the character and motivation, plus increased physical activity, is assured of achieving his goal.

Chapter 28

THE NUTRITIONALLY SOUND REDUCING DIET THAT GIVES YOU MORE VITALITY

by Eloise R. Trescher, R.D.

How many diets have you tried? Count them. If you're still heavier than you should be, something went wrong. Think about it, ferret out why! Be honest with yourself. Learn to know yourself.

Did you succumb to the temptation of the salted peanuts left over from last night's bridge game? If so, after the next party put them back in the jar as soon as the guests leave. Or was it the canister of cookies you made for the children? Move them to a place more difficult to reach—not from the children, from yourself. This may help you avoid eating unconsciously and perhaps surreptitiously.

There is no magic formula, no quick safe way to take off fat. But there is a way. If you know how many calories you should consume each day, and how many units of food chosen from the four food groups these include, you can lose weight with a balanced, nutritionally sound foundation diet.

A sound foundation diet, however, involves learning, moderation, consistency, persistence, implementation, and eternal vigilance. You may have to change your eating habits and food preferences. For example, accustom yourself to smaller portions; realize the absolute necessity of taking time to plan and prepare attractive, palatable, low-calorie meals; eat slowly (this increases enjoyment, cuts down on second help-ings); increase your physical activity.

A good breakfast is a *must*. If you have been passing up this meal you can *learn* to eat it. Get up 10 to 15 minutes earlier than usual if need be. You will start the day with more vim than with those few extra minutes of sleep. Remember that breakfast is the most important meal of the day in influencing your day's performance, and that of your husband and children. Take time to relax and enjoy it.

Each day your meals should include the basic four food groups (see page 129). Around these foods you should build your foundation diet. Change your eating habits, not for a day or a week, but forever. The calorie needs of men and women differ, and so do the amounts of food each requires. The 1,200-calorie pattern below is suggested for the healthy woman who wants to shed a few pounds. The 1,500-calorie diet would supply the basic needs of her healthy husband.

Now that you know the calories and the units of food you need, you must learn how much food equals a unit. The following lists show you the amount of food in one unit in the four different food groups. Buy a small scale that weighs in ounces, and a set of standard measuring cups. Use them until you carry a picture of the correct amounts in your mind.

Each amount listed is 1 MILK UNIT

1 cup skim milk, fresh or reconstituted nonfat dry milk
1 cup buttermilk (made from skim milk)
½ cup evaporated skim milk (an acceptable substitute for cream)

Each amount listed is 1 MEAT UNIT

1 ounce lean meat, fish, or poultry (cooked weight) no bone or fat
1 ounce Cheddar, Swiss, or other hard cheese (1 thin slice or 1-inch cube)
1 egg
5 oysters, shrimp, or clams (medium size)
¼ cup crab meat, cottage cheese, lobster, drained tuna, or salmon flake

Each amount listed is 1 FRUIT UNIT

*1 small apple—2-inch diameter
    or 1/2 medium*
1/2 cup unsweetened applesauce
1/3 cup apple juice unsweetened
*1/3 cup pineapple juice
    unsweetened*
1/2 cup diced fresh pineapple
1 small or 1/2 large pear
1/2 fresh mango—small
1/3 papaya—medium
2 fresh apricots—medium size
*1/4 honeydew melon—6-inch
    diameter or 1/8 melon,
    7-inch diameter*
*1/2 slice watermelon (with rind)
    1 inch thick*
*1 cup watermelon (without
    rind)*
2 fresh plums
10 cherries, Bing
12 grapes, large (24 small

*   seedless)*
1/2 small banana
1 medium nectarine
*1 orange (medium size)
**1/2 cup orange juice
    unsweetened (scant)*
*1/2 small grapefruit
**1/2 cup grapefruit juice
    unsweetened (scant)*
2 fresh figs
*1 cup tomato juice or V-8
*1 large tangerine
*1 cup strawberries
2/3 cup blueberries
1 cup blackberries
1 cup raspberries
**1/4 cantaloupe (6-inch
    diameter)*
1/4 cup prune juice unsweetened
1/4 cup grape juice unsweetened

*These fruits above are a rich source of vitamin C or ascorbic acid. Include at least one serving in your diet every day.

Fruit food units can also be canned fruits (packed in water), but you must remember always to count in the juice.

Canned fruit packed in water, 1 UNIT EACH

4 halves apricots and 1/3 cup juice
12 Royal Ann cherries and 2 tablespoons juice
2 halves peaches—no juice
2 slices pineapple and 2 tablespoons juice
3/4 cup strawberries including juice
1/2 cup blackberries including juice
1/2 cup fruit salad and 2 tablespoons juice
2 halves pears and 2 tablespoons juice
2 plums-prunes and 2 tablespoons juice
1/2 cup red raspberries including juice
1/2 cup blueberries

A bread unit, as you will read, takes on many forms.

Each amount listed is 1 BREAD UNIT

1 slice bread	⅔ shredded wheat biscuit
5 saltines	½ cup (scant) mashed or diced
3 large soda crackers	potato, peas, lima beans,
2 graham crackers	cooked rice, spaghetti,
3 Rye Krisps	noodles, macaroni, or grits
4–½ slices Melba toast	⅓ cup corn
3 triscuits	½ cup cooked dried peas,
½ matzo	lentils, or beans (scant)
½ cup any cooked breakfast	2½ level tablespoons flour
cereal	¼ cup yams
¾ cup dry cereal—flakes	½ English muffin
and puffed varieties	½ bagel
½ hamburger roll	

If you wish to substitute fruit for a bread unit, 1 bread unit equals 1½ fruit units.

Try to use no more than 1 cup of cooked vegetables at a meal, but in these Group A vegetables you may eat as much as you like raw.

GROUP A VEGETABLES

Asparagus	*Dandelion	*Peppers
*Beet greens	Dill pickle	Radishes
Brussels sprouts	Endive	Romaine
Cabbage	*Escarole	Sauerkraut
Cauliflower	Eggplant	*Spinach
Celery	*Kale	Squash, summer
*Chard	Lettuce	String or wax beans
*Chicory	Mushrooms	*Tomatoes—limit 1
Chives	*Mustard greens	serving a meal
*Collard	Okra	*Turnip tops
Cucumbers	*Parsley	*Watercress

*These vegetables above are a rich source of vitamin A. Include at least one serving in your diet every day.

GROUP B VEGETABLES

(½ cup of Group B vegetables equals ½ bread unit)

Beets	Onions	Rutabaga
*Carrots	Oyster plant	*Squash, winter
Kohlrabi	*Pumpkin	Turnips

*These vegetables above also are a rich source of vitamin A.

You may include without measuring

Water	*Pickles—sour or unsweetened*
Tea	*dill*
Coffee	*Mustard*
Vinegar	*Other spices*
Lemon	*Rennet tablets*
Mint and other herbs	*Unsweetened gelatin*
Clear broth or bouillon, fat free	*Artificial sweeteners*
Salt	*Cranberries*
Pepper	*Rhubarb*

Now knowing how many units of food you can correctly eat in a day, and what makes up these units, you can figure out your daily menus. Planning ahead makes meals more interesting, gives you a wider variety of foods and is certainly more fun. It's a game in a way, but quite a serious one, and you're sure to be a winner —by losing those extra pounds. You might find that you eat more than you do now, but if you discipline yourself to the right choices in the right amounts, you will lose weight.

Try this menu on a Sunday for a starter, a His and Hers menu based on this unit pattern; the recipes follow.

Hers *(1200 calories)*	**His** *(1500 calories)*
BREAKFAST	
½ grapefruit	*The same menu adding*
1 ounce kippers or	*½ cup cooked cereal with*
other meat unit	*part of 1 cup skim milk*
1 piece whole-wheat toast	*Café au lait (with remainder*
Café au lait	*of 8 ounces of skim milk)*
(use 8 ounces skim milk)	
LUNCH	
"Cream" of spinach soup,	*The same menu,*
Chef's salad	*adding an extra*
—low calorie dressing	*½ ounce each of cheese*
5 saltines	*and ham to the chef's salad*
Fruit cup	

Hers *(1200 calories)*	**His** *(1500 calories)*
DINNER	
Curried bouillon, again a cup	*The same menu plus two more*
Broiled filet mignon or any	*meat units and 1 more bread*
other selection from meat	*unit*
group	
Rice melange	
Broccoli spears	
Salad of apricots* (2 halves)	
and pear* (½)	
Lemon Snow pudding	
Demitasse	
*Canned, packed in water	

When preparing the recipes mentioned in the above menus, double when preparing for two, except in the case of Lemon Snow Pudding, and Chef's Salad, when more cheese and ham is necessary for the man's menu.

Recipes

"Cream" Soup. 1 cup skim milk; spinach or vegetables—lightly cooked or leftover; ½ teaspoon granulated chicken bouillon; seasoning to taste. Blend.

Fruit Cup. ½ orange; ½ banana (equals 1½ bread units); 12 grapes, seeded and cut in half.

Rice Melange. ½ cup cooked rice with sliced mushrooms, chopped celery, tomato, onion, green pepper, or parsley. Seasoning to taste.

Gelatin Dessert, as Lemon Snow Pudding. Soften 1 envelope Knox gelatin in ¼ cup cold water. Dissolve in ¾ cup boiling low-calorie soda of any flavor (in this case lemon flavor). Add 1 cup evaporated skim milk, artificial sweetener to taste, lemon juice (if needed) to taste. When almost set, fold in 1 egg white stiffly beaten. Pour into molds. Chill. Makes 2 servings.

To learn a safe way to attain a satisfactory weight takes time and patience. Moderation is the keynote, not total abstinence. For those who like a martini before dinner, *measure,* don't guess, the ingredients. Remember 1 ounce of rye, Scotch, bourbon, gin, rum, vodka, or brandy has 80 to 100 calories depending on the proof. So 2 ounces of one, in addition to your basic diet pattern, will not *prevent* your losing weight, but it may slow up your rate of loss.

The more one practices a habit, the more it becomes a way of life.

Milk Shake. 1 cup skim milk; flavor: almond, vanilla, chocolate, or rum extract, instant coffee, or 4 or 5 whole strawberries unsugared; artificial sweetner to taste; 2 ice cubes crushed. Blend.

Chef's Salad. Mixture of greens with ½ hard-cooked egg; ½ ounce slivered Swiss cheese; ½ ounce slivered ham; ½ ounce slivered turkey; low-calorie dressing; seasoning to taste.

BASIC REDUCING DIET

	Foods	**1200** *(women)*	**1500** *(men)*
Breakfast	*Fruit unit*	*1*	*1*
	Bread unit	*1*	*1*
	Meat unit	*1*	*1*
	Skim milk	*1 cup (8 ozs.)*	*1 cup*
	Tea or coffee	*free*	*free*
Lunch	*Meat unit*	*2*	*3*
	Vegetables	*free*	*free*
	Bread unit	*2*	*2*
	Skim milk	*1 cup*	*1 cup*
	Fruit unit	*1*	*1*
Dinner	*Meat unit*	*4*	*5*
	Vegetables	*free*	*free*
	Bread unit	*1*	*2*
	Fruit unit	*1*	*1*
	Skim milk	*1 cup*	*1 cup*

Snacks. Milk or fruit allowed at meals may be "saved" for between meal snacks. Skim milk may be used as cocoa, "cream" soup (see recipe), or a milk shake (see recipe).

Chapter 29

THE FOOD DIARY THAT TALKS BACK

by Eloise R. Trescher, R.D.

More than fifty years ago Frances Stern, founder and director of the Food Clinic in the U.S., at the Beth Israel Hospital in Boston, initiated the use of a daily food diary. Forty-five years ago the food diary was adapted for use in my nutrition clinic at the Johns Hopkins Hospital in Baltimore and is still in use. Today many clinicians, dietitians, nutritionists, pyschologists, pyschiatrists, and other investigators are using many variations of such records. Their effectiveness is undisputed. Such a record reveals important information about the patient and helps the patient learn about himself. The patient records the times of eating, the place, the circumstances and mood, the manner of eating, and the kinds and amounts of food and drinks. Through this he becomes conscious of factors that influence his weight (or disease) of which he was unaware. For example you should note:

When do you eat? Record the time and frequency of meals and snacks and the length of time spent in the process. Does the record reveal that meal times are given priority in planning the day's schedule or is food eaten on the run, sandwiched between activities? The latter method can result in rapid eating, ingesting larger quantities of food than needed and enjoying them less, as well as eating nutritionally inadequate snacks. Keep in mind that breakfast is the most important meal in the day. Allow time for it.

Where do you eat? Is it standing at the refrigerator or the kitchen counter? Or at the club, in the car, at the corner drugstore, a hamburger spot? Maybe it's at your desk, in a restaurant, on the terrace, in your garden, in the dining room or some other lovely and appealing room in your house. The atmosphere really matters. Meals should be relaxed. They are refresher times for the hours ahead. Approach those hours with equanimity.

Under what circumstances do you eat? Do you eat when you are really hungry, or when you are tempted by the sight or smell of food? Do you watch TV or read while eating? Do you eat when you are tired, angry, frustrated, nervous, anxious, or bored? Do you reward yourself with food when you have leisure time, feel happy and relaxed? Whatever your answer, find a satisfying substitute for that trip to the refrigerator. Do something creative, acquire a hobby, take a walk, go for a swim, engage in a sport. Just don't eat unnecessarily. Remember the old cliché: "Two seconds in your mouth, four hours in your stomach, and a lifetime on your hips!"

How do you eat? Do you eat rapidly from habit or to get that second helping? Stop it. Learn to eat slowly.

Do you chew thoroughly or do you wash food down with a beverage? Liquids with meals are fine—*provided* they are not used to expedite the swallowing process. Do you take large bites and gulp them down? If so, try eating in front of a mirror and see what big bites do to your face. If you are even a little vain you will take smaller bites.

Do you "chain" eat? Take a bite of food and lay down your fork or spoon between each bite. Eating slowly prolongs the pleasure of eating.

Do you eat surreptitiously? Remember calories do count, even when eaten secretly.

Do you choose the largest plate or glass? Use smaller ones; they hold less.

Do you eat outsized portions? Choose average ones.

With whom do you eat? Do you eat alone, with a friend, with a member of the family (which one)? Is the mealtime pleasant or a necessary chore? Make it pleasant.

THIS CHART WILL SUGGEST WAYS OF REDUCING CALORIES WITHOUT REALLY MISSING THEM				
You have been using	Calories	Use instead	Calories	Calories saved
1 cup—8 oz. whole milk	160	1 cup—8 oz. skimmed milk or buttermilk	90	**70**
Cheese, 1 oz. Blue, Cheddar, Swiss	105	Cottage cheese, 1 oz. creamed	30	**75**
		Cottage cheese, 1 oz. uncreamed	25	**80**
Hamburger, reg. 3 oz. Steak sirloin 6 oz. lean and fat	245 660	Hamburger, very lean Sirloin, lean only 6 oz.	185 345	**60** **315**
Pork chop thick 3½ oz. with bone, lean and fat	260	Pork chop 3½ oz. bone and fat discarded leaving 1.7 oz. lean	130	**130**
Beef or chicken pot pie	560	Broiled chicken, 6 oz.	230	**330**
Frankfurter 1, 2 oz.	170	Tuna (in oil) 2 oz. Tuna (in water) 2 oz.	110 75	**60** **95**
Sardines in oil 3 oz.	175	Crab, canned, 3 oz.	85	**90**
Lamb chop thick 4.8 oz. with bone, broiled lean and fat	400	Lamb chop, thick without bone and fat lean only 2.6 oz.	140	**260**
Fats—all kinds, butter, margarine, cooking and salad oils, 1 level tablespoon	125	1 level T whipped margarine	70	**55**
		2 level T sour cream	50	**75**
		1 level T jam, jelly, or honey	60	**65**
Waffle 1-2½ oz.	210	1 cup cooked oatmeal	130	**80**
Bagel 1 2 oz.	165	1 slice pumpernickel	60	**105**
1 Danish pastry without fruit or nuts	275	1 small plain doughnut	125	**150**
Hard roll 1⅔ oz.	155	4 saltines	50	**105**

What do you eat? Do you include adequate amounts of the four basic food groups in your diet every day (see page 129)?

A well-kept food diary will reveal all of these pertinent points. Others important to include are: *Sleep*—record your time of retiring and arising, the number of hours you need, and the quality of your sleep. Are you rested in the morning? Adequate rest is essential to our well-being. *Bowel movements*—are they satisfactory or unsatisfactory? If the latter, consult your physician.

Water intake should be recorded, as well as *exercise*, the usual and the unusual. The chief reason for unsuccessful weight-control programs is that persons want to see those pounds vanish rapidly. Be content with losing them as gradually as they were gained, and you are likely to accomplish your goal. We all overindulge from time to time, but when you do be moderate. The French author Camus put it this way: "Find indulgence in moderation." Weight control is self-control. Habits are not easily changed. Too much to eat and too little exercise are habits hard to break. Only permanent change in your eating habits and exercise pattern can bring permanent results.

Chapter 30

DIET SECRETS FROM FIVE WORLD-FAMOUS SPAS

1. THE GOLDEN DOOR

"A high-vitality life depends on high-vitality food," says Deborah Mazzanti, dynamic founder of the Golden Door, California's wonderful Japanese-style spa, whose low-calorie, low-cholesterol, natural foods diet for guests is beautiful to look at and taste. "Weight loss, however, is only partly due to decreased food intake; it is also due to exercise," says Mrs. Mazzanti, who serves on the President's Council on Physical Fitness and the board of the Menninger Foundation. She believes: "It's just as much fun to spend a calorie as it is to take one in." Increased movement at the Golden Door starts with an early morning walk-jog, goes on to exercise sessions that vary from warm-up exercises (Leonardo da Vinci's, inspired by his drawing of the Vitruvian Man), spot-reducing classes for specific problems, to water exercises in a warmed pool, yoga, and jazz dancing. They convert even the most slothful guests to Mrs. Mazzanti's maxim: "Eating allows you to live, but exercise allows you to live better."

The week (two for lucky ones) that guests spend at the Golden Door is not only a time for dieting and exercise, but a unique opportunity to get in tune with the body away from the stress of life, to renew oneself mentally and physically in an atmosphere of "disciplined serenity." Not exclusively a women's domain, there are eight scheduled men-only weeks and two weeks set aside for couples.

Diets are streamlined to the individual guest at the Golden Door by Mrs. Mazzanti and Chef Michel Stroot. It is an average 800 calories a day diet, but the counts swing from 500 to 1,100 calories, depending on one's personal diet requirements. Menus for a week and some of Michel Stroot's recipes can be found on page 223.

Deborah Mazzanti recommends the diet for one week a month maximum at home. If you wish to extend it, add two servings of whole grains (this could be ½ cup of whole grain cereal and a slice of home-baked bread) and peanut butter or an egg for added protein each day.

Mazzanti wisdom

What you learn from a week at the Golden Door is the importance of your own sense of well-being. The need for a balance between movement and rest. Movement comes first; rest is the reward. Exercise, divided into two periods each day—one for 10 minutes, one for· 30 minutes, should be tailored to suit your own system. If you're superbusy in the morning, exercise for 30 minutes—it will get you going; at the end of the day, exercise for 10 minutes more. If you tend to build up stress and tension during work, a 30-minute exercise slot at the end of the day will release tensions and help you unwind. In this case, schedule the 10-minute session the first thing in the morning.

During the day you build up carbon dioxide in your body; it adds weight and contributes to fatigue. If you exercise or breathe deeply at an open window, you expel the carbon dioxide and bring oxygen to the brain. The result is you feel refreshed.

Exercise to suit yourself, simply by walking if you wish, but at a fast pace and, to be effective, for at least 30 minutes.

Secret of small portions, small dishes

Everything at the Golden Door is served in tiny, pretty containers, diminutive lacquered bowls from Japan, and earthenware cocottes that hold just 1½ cups of liquid and give an illusion of a much larger portion. "Everything to do with eating is ritualistic and sensual," says Mrs. Mazzanti, "starting with the anticipation, the happiness of a family gathering, the sense of smell, taste, and texture when you eat."

Food served at the Golden Door by Chef Stroot is a constant delight to guests. Although low in calories, the skillful presentation and service give a feeling of leisurely satisfaction at mealtimes. Guests are encouraged to eat very slowly, and are served on individual trays from the kitchen. Lunch or dinner is of 45-minute duration; chopsticks are offered for eating salad, or if you prefer, a chilled fork. Nothing is provided to drink with a meal; "Liquids dilute the digestive juices you need for your food," says Mrs. Mazzanti who serves coffee, tea, or lemon water after the meal.

While you are trying to lose weight, Mrs. Mazzanti feels you should eat 10 percent of your total food intake at breakfast, 20 percent at lunch, and 70 percent for dinner (with a mid-A.M. and P.M. pickup—½ cup yoghurt or small tart apple and ½ ounce semi-skim-milk cheese to raise blood sugar). If you live alone, then you should have the main meal at lunch and something light, such as a large salad, in the evening. For a maintenance diet, switch to 20 percent for breakfast, 30 percent for lunch, and 50 percent for dinner.

Quick energy breakfasts

At the Golden Door, breakfast is served in bed on a tray after you've returned from an early morning walk on the hillside. "You simply need a small amount of food to raise your blood sugar and get you started on the day," says Deborah Mazzanti. Each day the tray has a different china, napkin, and place mat, a new nosegay of fresh flowers. Breakfast variations might include:

• A fresh peach, sliced and arranged with a strawberry or two for color. Tea with lemon.
• Breakfast surprise: peanut butter (about a teaspoonful) in center of peeled, cored pear half, tea with lemon.

• Yoghurt with a scattering of raisins and cinnamon; on the side, thin slices of orange; tea with lemon.
• Poached egg in its own little ramekin with, again, tea or coffee.
• Half a grapefruit with 6 black grapes, tea or coffee.
• Muesli with skim milk. To make it, combine chopped figs, rolled oats. Soak in water overnight. Next morning, stir in grated apple, hazelnuts, and cinnamon.

Low-calorie cooking tips
• Make salad dressings very strong in flavor, suggests Michel Stroot, then a little goes a long way. One cup salad dressing is enough for 30 salads.
• A teaspoon of honey will raise your blood sugar, give you vitality if you're tired.
• The Golden Door baked potato is just a jacket. Rub a baking potato with oil and bake. Cut it in half lengthwise, scoop out, leaving ½ inch potato on skin. Sprinkle with a few drops of oil, and return to a 400° oven for 20 minutes until crisp.
• *Golden Door Croutons* are toasted sesame seeds tossed over the top of a salad. *Vegetables* are served in big pieces to encourage crunching and munching. *Hot apple juice* with cinnamon and cloves is a wonderful cool day pickup. *Low-cholesterol omelettes* are made with 1 yolk and 2 egg whites, whisked up to a good froth before cooking. *Fresh herbs* for adding at the last minute or including in summer dishes can replace salt. *Grated cheese* makes a great thickener in sauces instead of flour. Use *ground mushrooms* to replace beef, 2 parts mushroom to 1 part ground beef cuts calories.
• To sauté the low-calorie way, use a heavy skillet and just rub it over with enough sesame seed, safflower, or sunflower oil to prevent the food from burning.

Nature in a glass
What a difference a day makes when you go on the Golden Door spa's new 24-hour liquid diet. Follow it on Monday and lose that pound or two put on after a festive

weekend; try it any day to launch a new low-calorie regimen. Deborah Mazzanti says, "It clears the system and gives
you an immediate psychological lift and an awareness of
feeling change in your body." Guests often use it to kick off a
diet week, and repeat it when they're in the midweek
doldrums. You can prepare the diet at home. All you need
are fresh fruits, vegetables, and nuts and a blender to whirl
them up in. You start with a breakfast glass of freshly
squeezed grapefruit juice, and sip a different drink every 2½
hours to keep blood sugar up and to give an energy boost. So
you don't feel "chew hungry," serve the drinks with a little
pot of sunflower seeds and 3 or 4 pine nuts, to be nibbled
slowly one by one. Drinks can be whipped in a jiffy and
should be served in 6-ounce glasses and sipped with a
demitasse spoon. The two almond milks, which supply
alkaline protein and amino acids, can be made at the same
time and the second serving stored in the refrigerator.

8 A.M. *Grapefruit Juice*
4 ounces freshly squeezed juice,
unsweetened, mixed
with 2 ounces water.
Calories 48
10:30 A.M. *Almond Milk*
12 whole almonds (or ½ ounce), blanched;
⅓ medium-sized, ripe banana; ¾ cup water;
4 ice cubes, dash vanilla and nutmeg.
Combine all ingredients and liquefy in
blender. Serve 6 ounces ice cold, over
ice. Makes 2 servings.
Calories 62
1 P.M. *Gazpacho*
1 medium tomato, peeled and diced;
¼ large cucumber, peeled and chopped;
¼ large green pepper, seeded; 1 slice onion;
2 sprigs parsley. Combine all ingredients
and liquefy in blender. Makes 6 ounces or more.

Calories 50

3:30 P.M. Pineapple-Cucumber Juice
3 ounces cucumber, peeled; 1 ounce fresh
pineapple; 2 sprigs parsley; 2 ounces
apple juice. Combine all ingredients and
liquefy in blender. Makes 6 ounces.
Calories 52

6 P.M. Almond Milk
See 10:30 A.M. recipe. The yield is sufficient
for both servings of almond milk
Calories 62

8:30 P.M. Carrot-Apple Juice
2 ounces apple juice; 2 ounces carrot juice;
⅓ apple, peeled. Combine all ingredients and
liquefy in blender. Makes 6 ounces.
Calories 69

⅓ ounce raw sunflower seeds mixed
with three or four raw pine nuts is
served with four of the six drinks.
Calories 59

CALORIE TOTAL FOR THE DAY: 579

Recipes

At the Golden Door, calorie counts for the day are
adjusted to each guest's specific requirements and vary
between 500 and 1,100 calories a day. The one-week menu is
modified for use at home where a low-calorie diet should
contain about 1,000 calories a day while you carry on normal
activities. Supplementary food and drinks, and snacks, are
served at the Golden Door between meals to boost energy.
For instance, 4 ounces either fresh orange or pineapple juice,
55 calories. A "cocktail," a low-calorie fruit slush that is
sipped through a straw, 25 calories, and raw vegetable

vegetable or cheese dip, about 30 calories, are served before dinner.

Soup Paysanne

When the soup is served as a main dish for lunch, Michel puts as many fresh vegetables into the soup as there are in the market, all cut Chinese-style. As a small side soup, only about 4 vegetables are needed. "It's impossible to get so many vegetables in such a small bowl!"

Ingredients
3 pounds bones—veal knuckle or chicken carcasses
Water
Vege Sal
Crushed peppercorns
4–5 bay leaves
2 teaspoons leaf thyme
2 celery roots, well washed and cut in quarters
2–3 leek tops, well washed and cut in large pieces
1 carrot, washed and whole
Parsley, chopped
2 onions studded with 4 cloves each
3 cups mixed vegetables, cut into small pieces. Choose from: spinach, broccoli, cauliflower, bean sprouts, bell peppers, celery, zucchini, leeks
Kikkoman soy sauce

Method
    In a tall 11-quart pot, put bones and fill the pot ¾ full of water. Bring to a boil, dump water out, reserve bones, and wash pot. (This is necessary with veal bones.)
    Fill pot again, add veal bones, and bring to a boil. Add Vege Sal, peppercorns, bay leaves, thyme, celery root, leek tops, carrot, chopped parsley, and onions and simmer for 4–5 hours.
    Skim the fat off the broth and defat as much as possible with paper towels.

Strain through cheesecloth.

Cut the fresh vegetables Chinese-style into small pieces on the diagonal. Add to the broth and bring it just back to the boil. Vegetables should still be tender-crisp. Season with soy sauce to taste. Makes about 2 gallons. *20 calories as side dish; 60 calories as a main dish.*

Tomatoes Oreganata

Ingredients
7–8 ripe tomatoes, peeled and cut in 6 pieces
Oregano
Vege Sal
Black pepper
¼ jar French mustard dressing (see recipe below)

Method
To peel tomatoes, cross bottom skin with knife and drop in boiling water for 2 minutes. Peel and put into stainless steel bowl, sprinkle with oregano, Vege Sal, and freshly ground black pepper.

Pour ¼ jar of French mustard dressing over tomatoes and marinate ½ day in the refrigerator. Serves 15. *50 calories per serving.*

French Mustard Dressing

Ingredients
2 full teaspoons Grey Poupon mustard
1 teaspoon black pepper
Scant ⅓ cup red wine vinegar
Scant ⅓ cup corn oil

Method
In an empty, clean Grey Poupon mustard jar put the mustard and freshly ground black pepper. Add red wine

vinegar to ½ way up jar. Add oil almost to the top. Shake well. *About 15 calories per teaspoon.*

Tomato Stuffed with Tiny Shrimp

Ingredients
4 ripe tomatoes
1 small garlic clove, minced
Olive oil
½ teaspoon fresh oregano
Salt
Black pepper, freshly ground
½ cup tomato juice
1 teaspoon fresh sweet basil
1 teaspoon fresh Italian parsley
1 teaspoon fresh chives
1 small zucchini, diced
½ pound spinach, chopped
8 ounces tiny bay shrimp, peeled and deveined
1 ounce Parmesan cheese, freshly grated
Bean sprouts

Method
Cut off tops of tomatoes and scoop out insides. Reserve tomato shells and tops and chop pulp.

In a large saucepan sauté the garlic in very little olive oil and add the chopped tomatoes, oregano, and salt and pepper to taste. Simmer for 15 minutes and add the tomato juice. Let simmer for another 20 minutes.

When sauce is cooked, add the herbs, vegetables, shrimp, and cheese and cook for 3–4 minutes. Stuff into the reserved tomato shells, sprinkle on a handful of bean sprouts, put the tops on, and serve immediately. Serves 4.
190 calories per serving.

Chicken Cocotte

Ingredients
2 whole chicken breasts, skinned, rib bones in (otherwise the meat will get too dry)
4 cups chicken broth, clear, strong, seasoned
Bay leaves
Fresh tarragon
Vege Sal
Italian herbs
½ cup carrots, peeled and sliced
½ cup turnips, peeled and sliced
½ cup cauliflowerets
½ cup green beans, cut into ½-inch pieces
½ cup snow peas, cut into ½-inch pieces

Method
Cut each chicken breast in half and place each in its own 1½-cup cocotte. Fill ¾ full with the chicken broth. Put a bay leaf in each, and season with fresh tarragon, if you have it, Vege Sal, and Italian herbs. Put on the lid and bake 35 minutes in a 375° oven.

Cook each vegetable in its own separate pot in a little bit of chicken broth until it is tender but still crisp.

When the chicken breasts are cooked, remove lids and add some of each vegetable to the cocottes. Serve more vegetables separately. Serve immediately. Serves 4. *200 calories per serving.*

Japanese Salad

All the vegetables are cut in very thin sticks.

Ingredients
Carrots
Zucchini
Cucumber
Bean sprouts

Celery
Watercress

Method
Arrange about ⅔ cup of the vegetables on a lettuce leaf. Spoon over a scant teaspoon of dressing. *50 calories per serving.*

Dressing

Ingredients
1 teaspoon lemon zest
1 tablespoon lemon juice
½ teaspoon soy sauce
½ teaspoon mustard
1 teaspoon wine vinegar
1 tablespoon salad oil
Salt to taste (optional)

Method
Put all the dressing ingredients into a blender and blend. *11 calories per teaspoon.*

Kabumushi

(Steamed, stuffed turnips)

Ingredients
5 small or medium turnips, washed and trimmed of top ½
    inch (save the tops) and bottom ¼ inch
1 medium eggplant, peeled and chopped finely
1 carrot, chopped
1 small onion, chopped
5 mushrooms, chopped
1 tablespoon oil
1 teaspoon soy sauce
1 teaspoon miso paste (soybean paste)
1 cup bean curd, mashed

Method

Steam the turnips for about 25 minutes or until tender. Let cool. Scoop out turnip flesh and reserve.

In a heavy pan sauté the eggplant, carrot, onion, mushrooms, in the oil until tender. Add turnip. Add the soy sauce, and miso paste. Add bean curd and stir together.

Fill the turnips with the vegetable mixture. Replace caps and steam for 15 minutes more. Serve with sesame sauce. Serve 1 turnip per person. *About 50 calories each.*

Sesame Sauce

Ingredients

2 tablespoons white sesame seeds, roasted
1 tablespoon miso paste
2 tablespoons soy sauce
3 tablespoons mirin (Japanese sweet wine) or light sherry
3 tablespoons sugar

Method

Whirl all the ingredients in a blender or beat with a mixer and serve with the turnips. Makes 1 cup. Spoon a very scant 1 teaspoon over stuffed turnip and replace cap.

Teriyaki Chicken

You may use the same method for steak or white fish.

Ingredients

3 chicken breasts, skinned and boned
1 small clove garlic, finely minced
1 small onion, finely minced
¼–⅓ cup soy sauce
1 teaspoon sake

Method

Marinate the chicken breasts for at least 18 hours in the garlic, onion, soy sauce, and sake.

Cut the chicken into small pieces and sauté quickly until tender. Assemble on small skewers. Serve chicken on individual hibachis. Serves 6. *80 calories per serving.*

Sauté Vincent

(Low-calorie mayonnaise)
Serve with cold poached salmon or as a dip for raw vegetables.

Ingredients
5 hard-boiled eggs
½ cup diet mayonnaise
1 egg yolk
½ cup lemon juice
Handful each parsley, basil, mint, chives, tarragon (all fresh)

Method
Remove yolks from 3 of the hard-boiled eggs and reserve for later use. Put mayonnaise in a blender with the 5 egg whites, 2 egg yolks, 1 uncooked egg yolk, lemon juice, and herbs and blend briefly until smooth.

Make just before using as the fragrance and texture will last only 1 hour. Serves 20. *20 calories per teaspoon.*

Lime Soufflé

Ingredients
10 egg yolks
1½ cups lemon juice, freshly squeezed, strained
1 teaspoon honey
1 envelope D-Zerta lime gelatin
1 envelope D-Zerta lemon gelatin
2 envelopes Knox unflavored gelatin
Boiling water
4 packages D-Zerta whipping cream
Zest of 1 lemon, grated
3 tablespoons Cointreau
18 egg whites

Method

In the top half of a double boiler put the egg yolks, lemon juice, and honey. Beat over boiling water until fluffy and remove immediately from heat. In a 1-cup measure put the 4 packages of gelatin. Add boiling water to make about ½ cup. Mix well to dissolve gelatin. Add cold water to make 1 full cup and pour into yolk mixture. Let cool over ice for about ½ hour and stir with a wire whisk occasionally so the bottom and sides will not set. The mixture should remain smooth.

Make the whipping cream according to package directions. In a heavy saucepan, add the grated lemon zest and enough water to cover. Boil for 1 minute. Strain through cheesecloth and Cointreau and bring to a boil again. Cook less than 1 minute. Let cool and add to the whipping cream. (Make sure whipping cream stays creamy and does not get stiff.)

Put the egg whites in a very large bowl and beat until they form stiff peaks, using an electric beater. Turn beater to lowest speed and immediately pour the yolk mixture into egg whites all at once. This part is critical—only 5 or 6 turns of the beater should be used to blend the 2 mixtures together. Fold egg white mixture ⅓ at a time into whipping cream. It should be light and fluffy.

Fit a 10-by-3-inch soufflé dish with a 4-inch foil collar with tape. Pour soufflé mixture into dish to within 1 inch from the top of the collar. Refrigerate the soufflé for about 4 hours to set. Serves 25. *75 calories per small slice.*

Fresh Fruit Sandwich

Serve 1 slice of each fruit cut ¼ inch thick. Stack them up and they look like a small pyramid.

Ingredients
3 ounces low-fat cottage cheese per person
¼ apple, grated
Cinnamon
1 scant tablespoon sunflower seeds

1 slice grapefruit, peeled
1 slice orange, peeled
1 slice pineapple, peeled
1 slice watermelon, peeled
1 slice kiwi, peeled
1 ounce dressing

Method for salad
Blend together with a rubber spatula the cottage cheese, grated apple, cinnamon, and sunflower seeds.

Layer the fruits with the largest slice on the bottom. Spread each with cottage cheese mixture. Top with slice of kiwi. Pour about 1 ounce of dressing on top. *190 calories per serving.*

Yoghurt Fruit Dressing

Ingredients
1 cup yoghurt
1 papaya, peeled
1 mango, peeled
1 cup strawberries, washed and hulled
1 teaspoon honey

Method
Whirl the yoghurt, papaya, mango, strawberries, and honey in a blender until smooth. Serves 30.

Veal Escalope Florentine

The seasoned spinach can also be tucked into an omelette or put on top of an oyster, baked.

Ingredients
1 pound spinach
Dash celery salt
Dash nutmeg
Fennel stalk, chopped

1 ounce Monterey Jack cheese, grated
Spice Island's Italian herbs
8–12 pine nuts
4 100-gram (3.6-ounce) veal escalopes
Few drops oil
Handful shallots, chopped
¼ cup dry white wine
Juice of ½ lemon
¼ ounce corn oil margarine

Method

Cook spinach fast for 2–3 minutes in ½-inch water in a large pan with 2 plates or a plate with a weight on top to weigh down the spinach. Cook just until wilted. Drain spinach and chop. Sprinkle with celery salt and nutmeg. Add just a little fennel.

Return spinach to pot over low heat and quickly stir in the cheese just until melted. Season with Italian herbs. Divide spinach into 4 portions, add 2–3 pine nuts to each, and wrap the veal escalopes around each portion.

Rub a few drops of oil in the bottom of a heavy skillet. Sauté veal quickly until brown, then cover skillet and put in preheated 350° oven for 10 minutes.

Remove veal to a heated platter. Over medium heat add shallots to skillet and sauté. Deglaze the skillet with the wine and lemon juice. Cook the sauce down. Stir in margarine. Return veal to pan for just a minute and serve immediately. Serves 4. *220 calories per 100-gram serving.*

Stuffed Zucchini, Chef's Style

You may substitute eggplant for zucchini in this recipe. The small Japanese eggplants are especially good to use. Can be reheated in a microwave oven.

Ingredients
12 zucchini, washed

Vege Sal
Oregano, dried
2 pounds mushrooms
1 large clove garlic
1 small onion
Pepper
Spice Island's Italian herbs
4 tomatoes, fresh or canned, chopped
4 ounces chuck steak, chopped and browned
1 ounce Parmesan, grated
3 ounces Monterey Jack cheese, grated
Parsley
Chives

Method

Cut zucchini in half lengthwise and crisscross flesh with a knife for easier cooking. Add to a large pot with ½ inch water and sprinkle the top with Veg Sal and oregano. Cover tightly. Cook on top of the stove over very low heat about 20 minutes, or in a 400° oven for 20–25 minutes. (Eggplants will take 35 minutes.) When cooked, scoop out center making sure to leave skin whole. Reserve skins and flesh.

Grate the mushrooms in a Cuisinart food processor or blender with the garlic and onion. In a skillet cook mushroom mixture very slowly and season with Vege Sal, pepper, Italian herbs. Add tomatoes, cook down.

Add the chopped chuck, Parmesan, and Monterey Jack. Mix well. Add reserved zucchini and cook down until firm.

Chop parsley and chives at the last minute and fold in. Fill the zucchini skins. Serves 12—one whole zucchini each. *200 calories per serving.*

Turkey Breast

Ingredients
1 12- to 14-pound turkey breast, skinned.

2 celery roots, peeled (reserve peels—they go in the pot to
help make the sauce)
2 white onions, studded with 4 cloves each
2 garlic cloves, peeled
Vege Sal
Bay leaf
Thyme
Summer savory
Peppercorns, crushed
2–3 ounces Neufchatel cheese
Juice of one lemon
Nutmeg, freshly grated
Chives, chopped

Method

Put the turkey breast in a large ovenproof pot with a tight
lid. Add the celery root and peels, onions, garlic. Season the
turkey with Vege Sal, bay leaf, thyme, summer savory, and
peppercorns. Cook at 400° for ½ hour, then 350° for 3 hours.
Never remove lid or the meat will dry out.

When cooked, remove turkey and keep it warm. Strain
and defat the broth (there will be lots of juice, but not much
fat).   Discard vegetables. Purée 2½ cups of broth in batches
in a blender.

Return the purée to the pan, add the Neufchatel, and
scrape the bottom of the pan. Add the lemon juice and a
grating of nutmeg. Adjust seasoning. Pour the sauce over the
turkey and sprinkle with chopped chives. Serves 30. *200
calories per 3-ounce serving.*

Fruit Slush
(Served as a "cocktail")

Ingredients
Strawberries, pineapple, peaches or any in-season fruit
Ice, cracked

Soda water, Fresca, or any diet soda
Kiwi slice or fresh mint for garnish

Method
    Use proportions of ⅓ fruit to ⅔ ice. Add the fruit and cracked ice to blender container and blend. Pour into tall glasses, thin with either soda or Fresca or any diet soda. Garnish with a slice of kiwi or fresh mint. Serve with a straw. *About 25 calories a 2½-ounce serving.*

Ginger Dressing
(For tossed green salads)

Ingredients
1 small clove garlic
1 tablespoon fresh ginger, chopped
Zest of 1 lemon without white pith
½ cup sesame seed oil
1 cup rice vinegar

Method
    Put all ingredients in the blender and blend to creamy stage. Makes 1½ cups. *14 calories per teaspoon.*

2. MAINE CHANCE

    Maine Chance, an oasis of green and flowers in the Arizona desert at Phoenix, provides a carefully balanced program of exercises, beauty treatments, and diet. The daily diet is high in protein and well-balanced with a total count of about 900 calories a day, including liquids. Guests who stick to the menu and combine it with three or four half-hour exercise sessions a day can lose several pounds a week.
    Protein in the form of meat, fish, or eggs is served twice a day in 350-calorie portions. The best-quality, simple, lean, roasted meats, broiled or baked chicken or fish are served on

attractive platters, guest honor-bound to take a carefully predesignated portion. Vegetables are always fresh and steamed to tender crispness. They are steamed slowly in the oven in a shallow baking pan with a little liquid and tight covering of aluminum foil until the liquid evaporates. Favorite vegetables: banana squash, mashed turnips, spinach rolled in tight, pretty balls. Salads are usually tossed sparingly with the Maine Chance dressing, a delicate and tangy blend of vegetable oil, greens, and egg yolks.

Dinner consists of a main course and a dessert, a low-calorie taste of something sweet—fresh or canned fruit, a sherbet or junket (skimmed milk with rennet) topped with a spot of apricot, papaya, or apple purée. On Saturday night, the close of a week, a graduation present comes, if you wish—a piece of one of Chef Joseph Bello's fragile cakes, served to gainers each day. After dinner, guests drink Sanka. Gainers, and there are usually one or two guests who wish to put on weight, are offered delectable desserts, snacks of sandwiches, and milk shakes during the day, extras such as baked jacket potatoes with their dinner, super-sized portions.

A week's menus to lose weight by, 900 calories per day

MONDAY

Lunch
Broiled lean hamburger
Stewed onions
Garden salad, Maine Chance dressing

Dinner
Roast rack of lamb au jus
(a serving of two small chops)
Banana squash
Strawberries and pineapple with maraschino

TUESDAY

Lunch
Shrimp (just 4) with deviled egg
Vegetable salad, Maine Chance dressing
Cooked vegetables with a
garnishing of chopped truffle and pimiento

Dinner
Broiled filet mignon
Garden carrots
Italian beans
Raspberry sherbet, yoghurt topping

WEDNESDAY

Lunch
Poached egg Florentine
Garden salad, Maine Chance dressing

Dinner
Roast prime ribs of beef
Mashed turnips
Steamed zucchini
Cantaloupe sherbet

THURSDAY

Lunch
Fresh fruit platter:
papaya, strawberries, grapes, pear, apple,
scoop of cottage cheese, yoghurt cream dressing,
Melba toast

Dinner
Roast breast of chicken
Spinach rolls
Creamed cauliflower
Junket with papaya purée

FRIDAY

Lunch
Broiled flounder
Coleslaw salad

Dinner
Roast rack of lamb
Steamed red cabbage
Green beans
Apricot mousse

SATURDAY

Lunch
Cheese soufflé
Garden salad, Maine Chance dressing

Dinner
Roast New York shell steak
Braised celery
Belgian carrots
Cake, torte

SUNDAY

Lunch
Mushroom omelette
Tossed salad, Maine Chance dressing
Canned diet fruit, with very little juice

Dinner
Roast spring chicken
Baked tomatoes
Green beans
Junket with apricot purée

One day's food and fitness program
7:30 A.M.
Breakfast
8:30 A.M.
Exercise—simple wake-up, warm-up bends and stretches; do them to music, it helps them flow. At home try towel exercises.
9 A.M.
Steam cabinet, sauna, or whirlpool bath—to cleanse and purify skin. At home, try Fluffy Milk Bath perfumed with Blue Grass by Arden.
10 A.M.
Massage—nothing beats the real thing for soothing aches, smoothing skin, but try massaging Body Cream into skin after bath for instant silkiness.
11 A.M.
Potassium broth—time for a poolside pickup, a hot vegetable broth served in a 4-ounce glass. Exercises—in the pool or tub, pushing and pulling limbs against water.
11:30 A.M.
Face treatment—cleansing, toning, and moisturizing refines skin in a gentle way. At home, try Arden's Bye-Lines Intensifying Mask, Velva Cream Mask, or Instantly Refreshing Mask.
12:30 P.M.
Scalp treatment—massage Eight Hour Cream briskly into scalp, brushing through. Leave for 24 hours. Hands and fingers, feet and toes, are treated, too. Try massaging your own feet and hands with Hand Cream and feel tensions slip away.
1 P.M.
Lunch
2:30 P.M.
Makeup class—spend half an hour at your own mirror and experiment to find the tools and tricks that work best for your face.

3 P.M.

Grapefruit juice, freshly squeezed into a 4-ounce glass; dilute with water if you wish.

3:30 P.M.

Exercise—half hour. There's a total of 90 minutes' exercising in a Maine Chance day. For additional exercises consult *Miss Craig's 21-day Shape-Up Program for Men and Women* (Random House, $7.95). A good habit to take home and keep up.

5 P.M.

Tea with lemon

6:45 P.M.

Cocktails—cranberry or tomato juice

7 P.M.

Dinner

Recipes

Maine Chance Salad Dressing

Ingredients
½ cup Wesson oil
½ cup salad oil
½ cup tarragon vinegar
1 teaspoon Vege Sal
1 teaspoon MSG
1 teaspoon dry mustard
1 teaspoon horseradish
3 egg yolks
1 bunch watercress, chopped
1 bunch parsley, chopped
6 shallots, chopped

Method
Put all ingredients in the blender to make a smooth,

creamy dressing. Add 1 large tablespoon ice water to dressing if it is too thick. Store in screw-top jar in refrigerator. Shake before serving. Makes 3 quarts. *9 calories per ¾-tablespoon serving.*

Cheese Soufflé

Ingredients
¼ cup butter, melted
¼ cup arrowroot
1 cup milk, heated
1 cup Cheddar cheese, grated
4 eggs, separated
¼ teaspoon cream of tartar
¼ teaspoon salt
Dash of cayenne or paprika

Method
In a saucepan mix butter with arrowroot. Cook over low heat 5 minutes. Add hot milk to the pan, stirring quickly with a whisk until smooth. Remove from heat, stir in cheese. When smooth like fondue, add egg yolks one at a time, stirring until smooth after each addition.

Beat egg whites with the cream of tartar in a large bowl with the salt until stiff. Gently fold cheese mixture into egg whites until well mixed. Add cayenne.

Grease 6 soufflé dishes 3 inches in diameter lightly with butter and fill ¾ full. Bake ½ hour at 350° on lower shelf of oven. Do not open door until time is up. Serve immediately. Makes 6 individual soufflés. *240 calories per serving.*

Vegetable Salad

Ingredients
½ cup carrot, cut in very thin strips
½ cup turnip, cut in very thin strips
½ cup green beans, cut in very thin strips

½ cup baby peas
½ cup cauliflower, broken into tiny flowerets
¼ cup Maine Chance dressing
Lettuce
Truffle
Pimiento
Beet

Method

Cook first 5 vegetables in separate saucepans in very little water until just tender, about 1 minute. Cool and drain. Toss vegetables with dressing.

Place vegetables on lettuce leaf. Garnish with diced truffle, pimiento, and strips of beet. Serves 4. *44 calories per serving.*

Raspberry Sherbet

Ingredients
4 cups raspberries, frozen or fresh
Low-calorie yoghurt for garnish

Method

Mash, press, whole fruit and juice through strainer with wooden mallet. Place in ice cream freezer. Serve with touch of low-calorie yoghurt on top. Serves 6. *65 calories per serving.*

Yoghurt Dressing

Ingredients
1 cup low-calorie cottage cheese
1 cup low-calorie yoghurt
2 tablespoons honey
2 tablespoons fresh lemon juice
1 tablespoon pineapple juice (optional)

Method
Whirl ingredients in blender until smooth. Makes about 2½ cups. *11 calories per tablespoon.*

Poached Egg Florentine

Ingredients
4 fresh eggs, lightly poached
2 pounds spinach, cooked, drained, chopped
4 thin slices toast, cut in triangles
Chopped truffle for garnish (optional)

Ingredients for sauce
3 tablespoons sweet butter
1½ tablespoons all-purpose flour
1½ cups milk
½ teaspoon salt
Dash nutmeg

Method
Arrange egg on top of spinach on each of 4 ramekins or plates. Place toast around. Top with white sauce and garnish with truffles.

Method for sauce
Melt butter in a saucepan, add flour, and cook 1 minute, stirring constantly. Lower heat, add milk, and stir vigorously until it boils. Cook and stir for about 5 minutes or until smooth and thick. Add salt and nutmeg. If too thick, add milk, then pour over eggs. Serves 4. *330 calories per serving.*

Potassium Broth

Ingredients
1 bunch carrots, unpeeled
6 parsnips, unpeeled
2 large onions
1 bunch parsley
3 leeks
1 whole stalk celery
10 quarts water
4 beef bouillon cubes, crumbled
3 egg whites, beaten
1½ tablespoons VegeSal

Method
Wash vegetables well. In large pot bring them to a boil in the water, simmer 3 hours. Add bouillon cubes, stir. Strain.

Add beaten egg whites to strained broth. Bring to a boil again to clarify. Add VegeSal. Strain through a cheesecloth or kitchen cloth. Serve hot with lemon slices. Keeps 1 week in the refrigerator. Do not freeze. Makes 5 quarts. *19 calories per 4-ounce serving.*

3. RANCHO LA PUERTA

At Rancho la Puerta, Deborah Mazzanti's world-famous health resort in Tecate, Mexico (just a two-hour drive away from her other health spa—the Golden Door), the food is hearty and vegetarian, but it's low-calorie, too. A balanced lacto-ovo vegetarian diet is served buffet-style three times a day. Guest scale portions to their individual diet goals. The suggested daily calorie count is 1,000. It comes in the form of fresh, natural foods and a wonderful dark stone-ground bread. It's a satisfying diet for most guests to lose weight by. Here are menus for a week, plus some of the Rancho's great recipes.

Rancho la Puerta's menus for à week

	Breakfast	Lunch	Dinner
Sunday	Half slice Tecate toast Individual casseroles of huevos Rancheros: 2 eggs poached with a sauce of tomatoes, onions, oregano, and basil Berries and yogurt sprinkled with date sugar	Hot spiced tomato soup Half avocado stuffed with pot cheese, celery, raisins Sesame bread sticks Fresh fruit	Sweet carrot soup Persian pancakes 1-ounce dish grated coconut and peanut butter Fruit salad 3-inch-square piece cheese cake
	Virtue Making Diet—The Golden Door's 1-day, 6-drink liquid diet (see House & Garden February, 1976)		
Monday	Half grapefruit Hot millet cereal with honey and skim milk	Small vegetable salad with alfalfa sprouts, sunflower seeds, and egg salad dressing Fresh fruit	Broth heated with fresh raw vegetables and sliced raw ginger. Greek olive and feta salad on a bed of chopped lettuce; oil, vinegar and oregano dressing. Stewed pears
Tuesday	Half slice Tecate toast Soft boiled egg Freshly grated red apple with skin, raisins, and cinnamon	Waldorf salad Rice-and-pine-nut-stuffed zucchini, oregano and tomato sauce Fresh fruit	Purée of spinach soup Red and white cabbage slaw Carrot-nut loaf Small baked banana with honey
Wednesday	Muesli: 1 ounce each oats and chopped dried figs soaked overnight in water, mixed with grated apple and 5-6 chopped hazelnuts. Served with skim milk	Fresh raw vegetable plate Assorted cheeses Baked apple stuffed with raisins and cinnamon	Sliced tomato and red onion salad; oregano, vinegar, and olive oil dressing Cream of peanut butter soup Broccoli soufflé Pineapple yogurt pie
Thursday	Egg poached in milk, margarine, salt, pepper Half slice Tecate toast Sliced orange with grated coconut	Cream of corn soup Raw vegetable sticks Yogurt and curry dip Spinach pie Fresh fruit	Tomato stuffed with guacamole salad—avocado mashed with celery and onion Cumino's soup Tostados with Salsa Mexicana Caramel slum custard
Friday	Papaya with lime Old-fashioned oatmeal sprinkled with bakers' bran, cinnamon, and raisins	Spring salad of sliced radishes, cucumbers, bell peppers mixed with yogurt and sprinkled with chives	Watercress and sliced raw mushroom salad; oil and vinegar dressing Gazpacho Cabbage rolls Grape pudding
Saturday	Grilled Monterey Jack cheese on half slice Tecate bread Fruit salad with toasted sesame seed and honey dressing	Caesar salad Eggplant Parmesan Fresh fruit	Mixed salad of lettuce, tomatoes, carrots; lemon and oil dressing Pinto bean soup Baked potato: baked, scooped out with only half the meat stuffed back in the skin after being whipped with cottage cheese, seasonings, and chives Apricot yogurt mold

Recipes

Tecate Bread

Ingredients
2 ounces yeast
4 cups warm water (105°–115° for dry yeast)
2 tablespoons honey
½ cup oil
7½–8 cups stone-ground whole wheat flour

Method

Place yeast in a very large bowl. Add warm water and stir. Blend in honey and oil. Add flour gradually while beating with an electric mixer. Keep adding flour until dough pulls off the beaters cleanly. Turn dough onto floured board and knead until it is no longer sticky. The dough is ready when it is silky and feels slightly bouncy, 8–10 minutes.

Divide dough in half, and roll each into a 12-by-15-inch oblong. Starting with the narrow end, roll up, jelly-roll fashion. Seal seam and fold each end over 1 inch. Place seam side down in 2 greased 9-by-5-by-3-inch loaf pans. Cover with a clean cloth and allow to rise in a draft-free, warm spot until double in bulk–about 1 hour. You can check to see if dough is ready by pressing the top with your finger. If a dent remains, the dough has risen enough.

Bake in a preheated oven (350°) 50–60 minutes, or until bread has a hollow sound when rapped on top and the loaves are well browned. (A teaspoon each of fennel and caraway seed can be added to dough for a different flavor.) Cool on racks. Slice each loaf into 22 slices. *105 calories per slice.*

To freeze, wrap in plastic wrap, pressing out as much air as possible. Can be kept frozen about 4 months.

Apple Snow

Ingredients
3 tablespoons lemon juice
1 tablespoon honey
4 tart, crisp apples, peeled and cored
3 ice cubes
Garnishes: mint, sliced lemon, or slivered candied ginger

Method
In a bowl, stir together the lemon juice and honey until honey dissolves. Grate the apples into the bowl and stir well. Chill until quite cold.

Crush ice in a blender and mix into apple mixture. Serve at once with a garnish of fresh mint, a lemon slice, or piece of candied ginger. Serves 4. *90 calories each serving.*

Salsa Mexicana

Ingredients
2 cups tomatoes, peeled, seeded, and finely chopped
⅓ green onion, chopped
⅓ cup coriander or parsley, chopped
1 clove garlic, minced
2 canned hot chili peppers, finely chopped (about 2 tablespoons)
1 teaspoon salt
¼ teaspoon dried oregano

Method
Combine all ingredients in a bowl and chill several hours. Serve this piquant relish with tostadas, over cottage cheese, or with guacamole. Makes about 2½ cups. *About 4 calories per tablespoon.*

Mexican Zucchini Casserole

Ingredients

2 tablespoons bread crumbs, toasted

2 eggs, separated

½ teaspoon salt

2 pounds (about 8 cups) zucchini, thinly sliced, steamed until just tender

Chili tomato sauce (see recipe below)

½ cup grated Monterey Jack cheese

2 tablespoons ripe olives, sliced

Method

Sprinkle crumbs over a buttered 9-inch-round casserole. In a bowl, beat egg whites until stiff; in another bowl, beat yolks with salt. Fold whites into yolks.

Layer half of the zucchini in the bottom of the casserole. Top with half the sauce, half the cheese, and finally half the egg mixture. Repeat, topping with the olives. Bake in a preheated 350° degree oven for 30 minutes, or until heated through. Serve hot. Serves 4 to 6. *125–185 calories per serving.*

Chili Tomato Sauce

Ingredients

1 tablespoon corn oil

¼ cup onion, chopped

1 canned green Ortega chili, washed, seeded, dried, and chopped

Salt to taste

1⅓ cups tomatoes, peeled, seeded, and chopped

1 teaspoon cumin seed, crushed

Method

In a skillet, heat oil and sauté onion and chili until onion is soft and transparent. Add salt, tomatoes, and cumin seed. Simmer for 10 minutes until sauce has thickened. Set aside.

Spanokopeta
(Spinach pie)

Ingredients for filling
2 tablespoons oil
½ cup green onions, including tops, chopped
2 pounds fresh spinach, stems removed, washed, dried, and chopped
⅓ cup parsley, finely minced
1 teaspoon dried dill
½ pound feta cheese, crumbled
5 eggs, beaten
2 partially baked pie crusts (recipe below)

Method for filling
In a large skillet, heat the oil and add the green onions. Sauté until tender.

Combine spinach, parsley, dill, feta, and eggs in a bowl. Mix and add to onions; blend well. Pour into partially baked pie crusts (or into 2 oiled 9-inch pie pans for soufflé-like crustless quiche). Bake in pre-heated 350° oven for 30–45 minutes until set. Makes 2 pies. Each serves 4. *330 calories per serving.*

Ingredients for crust
1½ cups whole wheat pastry flour
½ cup rye or soy flour
¼ teaspoon salt
3 tablespoons oil
3 tablesppons sesame tahini
3 tablespoons sesame seeds
⅓ cup water, or more
1 egg white (optional)

Method for crust

In a large bowl, add whole wheat and rye or soy flour and salt. Mix well. Add oil, tahini, and sesame seeds by hand, distributing thoroughly.

Add water, a little at a time, kneading until dough is workable. Roll out on a floured board and place in pie pans.

Brush with egg white (if desired) and prick bottom and sides with a fork. Bake in a preheated 400° oven for 8 minutes.

Cool and fill. Makes two 9-inch crusts. (Top crust may be used if diet allows. If so, two crust recipes will be needed.)

Grape Pudding

Ingredients
1 tablespoon brown sugar
2 cups pure Concord grape juice
3 tablespoons arrowroot
⅛ teaspoon ground cinnamon
⅛ teaspoon ground cloves
1 teaspoon Ouzo, Pernod, or ¼ teaspoon anise extract
Orange slices
Chopped walnuts

Method

In a heavy saucepan, dissolve sugar in 1½ cups grape juice and bring to a boil. Mix remaining juice with arrowroot in a small bowl and slowly add it to the boiling juice, stirring constantly. Add cinnamon and cloves and cook until thick. When thickened, stir in Ouzo, Pernod, or anise extract and remove from heat. Cool.

Pour into 4 wine glasses and chill. Garnish each with an orange slice and 1 teaspoon chopped walnuts. Serves 4. *123 calories per serving.*

Sweet Carrot Soup

Ingredients
½ medium-size onion, chopped
3 tablespoons margarine or corn oil
½ teaspoon curry powder
¼ teaspoon coriander (optional)
½ teaspoon brown sugar or honey
3½ cups vegetable stock, boiling
¾ pounds carrots, scraped and diced
4 teaspoons flour
¼ cup low-fat milk
1 egg yolk
Chopped chives

Method
In a deep skillet, sauté onion in 2 tablespoons of the margarine or oil. Add curry and coriander and cook another minute. When fragrant, add sugar, stock and carrots. Simmer, covered, until carrots are quite tender. Purée and reserve.

Heat remaining margarine or corn oil in a large saucepan, and add flour, stirring until smooth. Slowly pour in milk. Cook, stirring, over low heat until thick. Remove from heat and beat in egg yolk. Add carrot purée and return to heat, gradually heating to just below boiling point. Garnish with chives and serve at once. Serves 6 to 8. *80–100 calories per serving, depending on the size of the serving.*

Pinto Bean Soup
(Sopa de frijol a la olla)

Ingredients
1 tablespoon oil
2 green onions, cut in 1-inch lengths
2 cloves garlic, minced
1 medium green pepper, coarsely chopped

¼ cup tomato peeled, seeded, and chopped
1 cup cooked pinto beans (recipe below)
3 cups pinto broth (recipe below)
1 teaspoon coriander or parsley, finely chopped
Salt to taste
Garnishes: ¼ cup coriander, chopped; ¼ cup tomatoes, peeled, seeded, and chopped; ¼ cup onions, chopped; ½ cup Monterey Jack or Romano cheese, grated

Method

In a large saucepan, heat oil and sauté green onions, garlic, and green pepper until slightly soft, 3–5 minutes. Add tomatoes, pinto beans and broth, coriander or parsley, and salt to taste. Bring to the boil and boil briskly, uncovered, 10 minutes. Makes 4 large servings. Garnish at the table with the coriander, tomato, onion, and grated cheese. Each serving is a full meal. *240 calories each.*

Ingredients for pinto beans and broth
1 pound pinto beans
3 garlic cloves
1 gallon water
Salt to taste

Method for pinto beans and broth

Wash beans. Put them in a large kettle and add garlic and water. Bring to the boil and simmer 1 hour. Add salt to taste and simmer another hour. Strain beans, reserving the water. Use beans and cooking liquid for the bean soup. *¼ cup beans, 25 calories.*

Persian Pancakes

Ingredients
1 egg, beaten
1 cup skim milk
Dash salt

1 cup whole wheat pastry flour
1 tablespoon baking powder
Cheese filling (recipe below)
Sauce (recipe below)

Method

Mix egg and milk in a small bowl. Put salt, flour, and baking powder in a bowl and stir well. Slowly add dry mixture to milk mixture beating briskly until smooth. Pour about ¼ cup batter for each pancake onto a lightly oiled medium-hot griddle or heavy pan. Turn when pancake bubbles, cook other side, remove, cool. Spoon 2 heaping tablespoons of filling on each pancake, roll, place in a casserole. Heat in a preheated 250° oven 10 minutes. Serve topped with warm sauce. Makes 8 pancakes. *180 calories each with cottage cheese; 200 calories if filled with ricotta.*

Ingredients for filling

1 cup ricotta cheese or low-fat cottage cheese (if cottage cheese, press through a sieve)
¼ cup raisins
1 teaspoon cinnamon
2 tablespoons brown sugar

Method for filling

Combine ingredients thoroughly.

Ingredients for sauce

1¼ cups apple juice or cider
3 tablespoons arrowroot or cornstarch
3 tablespoons pure maple syrup

Method for sauce

Heat 1 cup juice or cider in a small saucepan. Mix arrowroot or cornstarch with the remaining juice. Stir until smooth. Add to the boiling juice slowly. Stir constantly, cook until thick. Remove from heat, stir in syrup. Serve hot.

Apricot Yoghurt Mold

Ingredients
2 tablespoons unflavored gelatin
½ cup pineapple juice
2 cups dried apricots, simmered in 3 cups water for 15 minutes, then drained
2 tablespoons lemon juice
1 tablespoon lemon zest, finely grated
2 eggs, separated
2 cups plain yoghurt
Garnishes: unsweetened, grated coconut; chopped almonds; or strawberrries

Method
In a small saucepan, add gelatin and pineapple juice. Heat gently and stir until gelatin is dissolved. Remove from heat.

In blender, purée apricots, lemon juice, zest, and egg yolks. Turn blender to low and add gelatin mixture. Cool in refrigerator until slightly jelled, about 15 minutes.

In a bowl, beat egg whites until stiff. Combine gelatin mixture thoroughly with yoghurt in a large bowl, and fold in egg whites. Pour into an 8-cup mold or individual dishes. Chill. Garnish with unsweetened coconut, chopped almonds, or strawberries. Fresh fruit may be substituted for dried apricots for a lower calorie count. Serves 6 to 8. *285–368 calories.*

4. THE GREENHOUSE SPA

For anyone in your family who wants to lose weight, it's almost painless if the food is delicious and beautiful at the same time. Food consultant Helen Corbitt, who believes the appearance of food is almost as important as the taste, planned this week of menus and recipes based on those she does for guests at The Greenhouse, the luxury spa in

Arlington, Texas, owned and operated by the Great South-west Development Corporation. "Learn to know which foods are lower in calories and eat smaller portions of everything," says Miss Corbitt, who chooses food that is full of vitamins and minerals, but low in carbohydrates and fats. "Balance your diet by including all the food groups: milk, meat, vegetables, bread, and cereals. You can take off pounds if you reduce the calories it takes to maintain your ideal weight."

Corbitt's slimming secrets

—"Sit down and think about all the things that go into making a meal attractive, and don't try to plan it in the supermarket.

—"Men and children respond to texture and flavor, which go into the makeup of attractive food, and they will be unaware of the fact that they are eating a lower-calorie but satisfying meal.

—"Follow the old-time nutrition guides of lean meats, poultry or fish, fresh fruits and vegetables, skim milk instead of whole, little or no sugar (there is no biological need for it), whipped vegetable oil margarine in place of butter, especially if you are cholesterol minded, and less salt.

—"No snacks unless they are fresh fruits or vegetables. Cook vegetables carefully to insure their vitamin content.

—"Take an extra few minutes to make food look good: thinly sliced meat really looks better than thick; watercress and parsley give an extra spark of color; vegetables look more appetizing when they're thinly slivered.

—"Anyone dieting for cosmetic reasons should accept the fact that a low-calorie diet alone will not do much for inches, just as exercise alone does not do much for weight reduction, but you do need both!

—"Breakfast is a personal thing for most people, but I recommend fresh fruit or juice, 1 egg or 2 ounces cottage cheese, and 1 very thin slice dry toast to give a good start for the day.

—"A demitasse cup of soup is a good pick-me-up. Keep one of beet yoghurt soup, for instance, in your refrigerator.

—"Any salad dressing can be cut down with water to decrease calories. It is only the flavor you want anyhow, and a teaspoonful on a small salad is enough. Everyone has a tendency to overdress a salad.

—"Use grated citrus fruit peel to flavor vegetables. Grated vegetables such as carrots, beets, and radishes add both color and flavor to vegetable dishes."

The Greenhouse Spa's Menus for a Week

LUNCH	DINNER
SUNDAY	
Fresh Strawberries with Puréed Raspberries	*Beet Yoghurt Soup*°
Piperade with Canadian Bacon°	*Singapore Turkey with Natural Juices*
Popovers	*Baked Cranberries with Orange*
	Fresh Green Beans with Scallions
	Parslied Mashed Cauliflower
	Fresh Spinach and Mushroom Salad
	Cold Lemon Soufflé made with skim milk °
MONDAY	
Half a Papaya filled with Cold Shrimp, Grated Coconut, and Fresh Lime Juice	*Essence of Tomato Soup*
Very Cold White Asparagus	*Broiled Flank Steak Marinated in Soy Sauce and Fresh Ginger*
	Thinly sliced White Turnips, Heavily Parslied
	Zucchini Cups Filled with Sautéed Mushrooms
	Celery Salad with Mustard Dressing°
	Steamed Fresh Pears, Red Wine Syrup
TUESDAY	
Julienne of Turkey (leftovers) in Aspic on Boston Lettuce	*Rosemary Broiled Leg of Lamb*
Slices of Fresh Pineapple	*Eggplant Provençale*°
	Sliced Brussels Sprouts with Grapes
	Romaine and Shredded Radish Salad, Vinaigrette Dressing
	Apricot Sponge°
WEDNESDAY	
Crudité Salad with Sherry French Dressing	*Jellied Watercress Soup*
Small Scoop Cottage Cheese or Thin Slice Leftover Lamb	*Tandoori Roast Chicken*°
Baked Cinnamon Grapefruit	*Savory Fresh Spinach*
	Sautéed Little White Onions and Mushrooms
	Chunky Iceberg Lettuce with Diced Hot Broiled Fresh Pineapple
	Coffee Pots de Crème

LUNCH	DINNER
THURSDAY *Individual Cheese Custard, baked in shallow casserole (a nice Sunday night supper dish also) Zucchini and Cherry Tomatoes with Sesame Seeds° The Greenhouse Orange*	*Chopped Vegetable Salad,° Pear Vinegar Dressing° Peppered Top Butt of Beef Baked White Squash, Paprika Stir-Fried Spinach with Grated Beets Ricotta Cheese Pie with Puréed Strawberries°*
FRIDAY *Individual Carrot Pudding Zucchini Fan with Parmesan Honeydew Melon Boat*	*Cucumber Boat Filled with Diced Tomatoes and Celery, Green Herb Dressing Fillet of Sole Roulade with Fresh Salmon and Dill Sauce, Lemon Cup filled with Capers° Tomato filled with Puréed Green Beans Asparagus with Grated Orange Peel Three Fruit Sherbet*
SATURDAY *Bouillabaisse ° Romaine, Red Cabbage and Grapefruit Salad, Sherry French Dressing*	*Marinated Fresh Artichoke Cinnamon and Lemon Roasted Leg of Veal, Natural Juices ° Broccoli Soufflé Celery and Snow Peas Red and Green Pepper Salad Stained Glass Window Pie*

Recipes

Beet Yoghurt Soup
(In a demitasse)

Ingredients
1 cup cooked beets, finely chopped
1 hard-boiled egg white, chopped
½ cup cucumber, finely chopped
4 green onions, finely chopped
¼ teaspoon dill weed
1 cup yoghurt
½ cup shrimp, finely chopped (optional)

2 tablespoons parsley, finely chopped
½ cup ice water
Salt and pepper
Lemon slices
Ice cubes

Method
Blend all ingredients, chill, and serve in cold cups with slice of lemon floating on top and with an ice cube for each cup. Serves 8. *45 calories per serving.*

Cold Lemon Soufflé

Ingredients
2 teaspoons unflavored gelatin
1¼ cups cold milk
2 egg yolks
¼ cup lemon juice
Pinch of salt
2 teaspoons sugar substitute (or more)
1 teaspoon grated lemon peel
¼ teaspoon lemon extract
2 egg whites

Method
Soften gelatin in milk. Mix egg yolks, lemon juice, salt, and sugar substitute. Cook over hot water with the gelatin mixture until thickened. Remove, cool, add peel and extract. Beat egg whites until stiff, fold into the lemon mixture. Pour into mold and chill. Serves 8. *50 calories per serving.*

Mustard Dressing

Ingredients
1 cup plain yoghurt
1 heaping tablespoon Dijon mustard
Few drops of lemon juice

Method

Mix ingredients and serve with any salad. *140 calories per cup; 8½ calories per tablespoon.*

Apricot Sponge

Ingredients
1 tablespoon unflavored gelatin
1 cup skim milk
2 eggs separated
1 cup puréed water-packed apricots
1 teaspoon sugar substitute
½ teaspoon almond extract
Optional: soft custard, puréed fresh strawberries.

Method
Dissolve gelatin in milk. Beat egg yolks until lemon yellow and add to milk. Heat over hot water until gelatin is dissolved and mixture thickens. Remove, cool, and add apricots, sugar substitute, and almost extract. As it begins to congeal, fold in stiffly beaten egg whites. Pour into mold and chill. Unmold and serve with soft custard or puréed fresh strawberries if you wish. Serves 6. *59 calories per serving.*

Tandoori Roast Chicken

Ingredients
3 cups plain yoghurt
6 cloves garlic, crushed
1½ tablespoons fresh ginger, grated
¾ cup lime juice
2 tablespoons coriander, ground
1 tablespoon cumin
1 teaspoon cayenne pepper
1 teaspoon powdered anise
2 ¾-pound broiler chickens
Lime wedges
1 onion, sliced and steamed

Method

Mix yoghurt, garlic, ginger, lime juice, and spices. Rub chickens inside and out with mixture. Place in a bowl and pour rest of marinade over. Cover and marinate in the refrigerator for 24 to 48 hours. Turn chickens at least once if not completely covered. Preheat oven to 375°. Remove chickens from marinade, place in a pan, and roast until done, about 1 hour. Baste with the marinade. Disjoint and serve with wedge of lime and onion. Do turkey the same way. Serves 8. *Half chicken, 185 calories; ¼ chicken, 93 calories.*

Ricotta Cheese Pie

Ingredients
2 tablespoons lemon juice
1 tablespoon unflavored gelatin
½ cup hot skim milk
1 teaspoon orange peel, grated
2 eggs, separated
2 teaspoons sugar substitute
2½ cups soft ricotta cheese
1 cup crushed ice
Puréed fruit, optional

Method

In a blender add juice and sprinkle gelatin on top. Add hot milk, orange peel, egg yolks, sugar substitute, and cheese. Whip at high speed for 2 minutes. Add ice and run at high speed until well blended. Beat egg whites until stiff. Fold into mixture. Chill in oblong pan or pie tin until firm. Serve next day. Cut in wedges or squares and serve with puréed fruit.

When strawberries are in season, cover with whole berries and pour puréed berries over and make in layer-cake pans. Serves 12. *90 calories per serving.*

Piperade with Canadian Bacon

Ingredients
4 teaspoons whipped margarine
1 green pepper, thinly sliced
1 white onion, thinly sliced
2 tomatoes, peeled, seeded, sliced
Salt and pepper
4 eggs
4 tablespoons skim milk
Grated Parmesan cheese
Chopped parsley or chives
1 clove garlic, optional
Canadian bacon

Method
Melt two teaspoons margarine, add vegetables, and cook at medium heat until just tender. Season with salt and pepper. Keep warm. Melt rest of margarine. Mix the eggs and skim milk, with a pinch of salt and pepper. Add to the margarine and cook over low heat until soft and moist, not solid. Spoon the vegetables on a platter to form a ring, add the eggs and sprinkle a little Parmesan cheese over. Sprinkle with the parsley or chives. A garlic bud may be added to the vegetables if you wish, but remove before serving, and never before 10 A.M. Surround with broiled thin slices of Canadian bacon. Serves 4. *119 calories per serving. Canadian bacon, 79 calories per 1-ounce slice.*

Eggplant Provençale

Ingredients
1 eggplant peeled and sliced in 1-inch-thick slices
2 cups fresh tomatoes, peeled, seeded, and chopped
1 cup onion, chopped and cooked
1 clove garlic, minced
Pinch of thyme

4 tablespoons parsley, chopped
Salt and pepper
Parmesan cheese

Method

Put eggplant slices on a lightly oiled pan and broil about 8 minutes. Set aside. Sauté remaining vegetables and herbs and cook until thickened. Season with salt and pepper. Pile on top of the eggplant. Sprinkle with cheese and bake in 350° oven until hot and golden brown. Serves 8. *31 calories per serving.*

Zucchini and Cherry Tomatoes with Sesame Seeds

Ingredients

2 or 3 zucchini
1 tablespoon whipped margarine
2 tablespoons onion, finely chopped
½ clove garlic, finely chopped
¼ cup cherry tomatoes, cut in half
Salt and freshly ground pepper
1 tablespoon sesame seeds, toasted
2 tablespoons parsley, finely chopped

Method

Wash and slice squash on the bias. Blanch with boiling water for 1 minute. Drain. Melt margarine, add onion and garlic. Sauté on medium-high heat for 1 minute. Add squash. Cover and cook 2 minutes. Add tomatoes, cover and cook 30 seconds. Season, add sesame seeds and parsley. Toss gently and serve. Serves 4. *50 calories per serving.*

Chopped Vegetable Salad

Ingredients

1 head romaine, finely chopped
¼ cup very crisp bacon, finely diced

2 tablespoons Roquefort cheese
3 tomatoes, peeled, seeded, and finely diced
1 avocado, peeled and diced
2 hard-cooked egg whites, chopped finely
1 tablespoon pimiento

Method
    Mix ingredients well and refrigerate. Serves 8. *90 calories
per serving.* Toss with pear vinegar dressing (recipe below).

Pear Vinegar Dressing

Ingredients
¼ cup pear vinegar
½ cup safflower oil
1 teaspoon lemon juice
1 clove garlic, crushed
Salt and freshly ground pepper

Method
    Mix ingredients well and let stand a few hours before
using. Serves 8. *42 calories per tablespoon per person.*

Bouillabaisse

Ingredients
1 white onion, sliced thinly
2 leeks, sliced thinly
2 fresh ripe tomatoes, peeled, seeded, and chopped
1 quart water or fish stock if on hand
1 rib celery
1 carrot
Few sprigs of parsley
1 piece of orange peel
1 or more cloves garlic, crushed
1 bay leaf
Pinch saffron

1 cup clam juice
¼ cup dry white wine
½ pound uncooked red snapper cut in 1-inch squares
¼ pound uncooked haddock or cod, cut in 1-inch squares
8 clams in shell
½ pound uncooked shrimp or lobster tail or both
Salt and pepper
Pinch of cayenne
Parsley, chopped

Method

In a large pot, mix the first 11 ingredients and simmer at medium heat until onions and leeks are tender, about 30 minutes. Add clam juice, wine, snapper, and haddock or cod. Cook for 10 minutes. Add clams and shrimp or lobster or both and cook until clams open. Season with salt, pepper, and cayenne. Remove celery, carrot, garlic, and parsley. Add chopped parsley when served. Serves 4. *185 calories per serving of 2 clams, 2 shrimp, 2 1-inch squares fish, a little stock, and vegetables.*

Fillet of Sole Roulade

Ingredients

1 thin slice fresh salmon, cut in 4 pieces
4 fillets of sole, 2–3 ounces each
½ cup white wine
½ cup water
4 slices lemon
Arrowroot
1 teaspoon dill weed
Salt and white pepper
Lemon cups
Capers

Method

Lay the salmon on top of the sole and roll. Fasten with a

toothpick and poach covered in half water, half dry white wine, slices of lemon, about 10 minutes or until fish flakes. Strain liquid, slightly thicken with arrowroot, 1 teaspoon to 1 cup liquid. Add dill weed and season with salt and white pepper to taste. Garnish with lemon cups filled with capers. Serves 4. *96 calories per serving.*

Cinnamon-and-Lemon-Roasted Leg of Veal, Natural Juices

Ingredients
1¾ pounds veal for roasting
1 teaspoon salt
¼ teaspoon white pepper
½ teaspoon cinnamon
Grated rind of 2 lemons
Juice of 2 lemons
½ cup dry white wine

Method
Preheat oven to 350°. Rub veal with salt, pepper, and cinnamon and roast for 1 hour. Add rind and juice of lemons to pan and baste with white wine. Basting frequently, roast for 1 hour more or until a fork thrust into the meat comes out easily. Slice thin and serve with pan juices. Serves 10 to 12. *225 calories per serving of 2 ounces cooked veal.*

5. EUGENIE-LES-BAINS

If you were a guest at the famous French spa, Eugénie-les-Bains, you would enjoy these delicious menus and recipes as part of your special health regimen. They are the creations of Michel Guérard, whom many now call the most inventive chef in France. Here he shares with you his secrets and principles of successful low-calorie cooking.

A few principles of Michel Guérard
• Low-calorie food must taste so good and look so good that psychologically you never feel deprived but mentally prefer it. In time, you well may.
• You can have haute cuisine with a low calorie count—approximately 1,000 calories a day.
• A feast for the eye is an important element of nourishment. Every Guérard dish is a stunning composition. Automatically you slow down to contemplate and admire it. Eating slowly is one key toward satisfaction.
• The judicious use of a blender gives a creamy texture without resorting to cream.
• You need sharp knives, a blender, and a Teflon pan.
• Vegetables are sliced and diced so fine, they can be cooked in a few turns around a Teflon pan without the addition of any fats.
• Sauces are one of the delights of French cuisine and are featured in Guérard's Eat Yourself Slim regime. As thickening agents, use puréed vegetables or low-calorie white cheese. (In France, Taillefine. In America, farmer cheese, diet cream cheese, ricotta, yoghurt cheese.)
• In this lighter way of eating, there are no potatoes, rice, noodles, or bread.
• Every lunch and dinner is a three-course meal, ending with a dessert made with an artificial sweetener.
• The Tisane d'Eugénie—an infusion of five health-giving herbs and plants—is served several times a day. At breakfast. Before lunch. Before dinner. The tisane is a natural diuretic. It is presented with the charm of a planter's punch, in tall glasses garnished with a slice of apple, a slice of orange, a grape, a chunk of pineapple, a sprig of fresh mint.
• Meats can be grilled without fat or oil by giving them a fast dip in water. The evaporating moisture will keep them from sticking to the pan.
• To banish hunger pangs for familiar but fattening foods, Guérard offers a variety of pleasurable taste surprises and the excitement of totally new culinary inventions.

• Seasoning is vital—salt, pepper, and generous doses of fresh herbs. Much of the sensory excitement comes from the seasoning.

Cuisine Minceur Lunch
Onion Tart
Grilled Escalopes of Veal
with Tomatoes Provençale
Assortment of Sherbets
with fruits

Onion Tart

Ingredients
1 cup plus 2 tablespoons water
¾ cup carrots, very finely diced (same size as peas)
5⅔ cups onions, sliced very fine
1 cup mushrooms, very finely diced (same size as peas)
4 tablespoons green peas, cooked
Salt and pepper
1 green cabbage, leaves separated and stems cut away
7 tablespoons skim milk powder
3 eggs, beaten
1 tablespoon parsley, chopped
1 tablespoon chervil, chopped
½ teaspoon tarragon, chopped

Method
Preheat oven to 200°. In a Teflon pan add 2 tablespoons of water, carrots, and onions and sauté for 10–15 minutes; add mushrooms and peas for the last few minutes. Salt and pepper to taste and set aside.

Boil cabbage in salted water 8–10 minutes and drain. Line six 4-inch individual tart pans with leaves and reserve leftover ones. Fill pans with vegetable mixture and set aside.

Mix milk powder with 1 cup water and add eggs, parsley,

chervil, and tarragon and mix well. Pour mixture over vegetables and cover each with a cabbage leaf.

Bake for about 45 minutes. Unmold and serve hot. Serves 6. *123 calories per serving.*

Grilled Escalopes of Veal with Tomatoes Provençale

Ingredients
6 tomatoes, cut in half crosswise
Salt and pepper
1 teaspoon garlic, chopped
6 thin escalopes of veal
Water flavored with 1 garlic clove, crushed
2 tablespoons parsley, chopped

Method
Preheat oven to 350°. Sprinkle each tomato half with salt, pepper, garlic, and parsley and bake for 10 minutes.

Season veal with salt and pepper, and dip in garlic water. Broil 1 minute on each side. Serves 6. *195 calories per serving.*

Raspberry Sherbet

Ingredients
2 cups raspberry pulp, sieved
Juice of 2 lemons
1 cup water
Artificial sweetener to taste

Method
Combine raspberries, lemon juice, and water. Sweeten to taste, stirring until sweetener is dissolved. Freeze in an ice-cream maker. Serves 6. *31 calories per serving.*

Melon Sherbet

Ingredients
½ cup skimmed milk
2 cups cantaloupe melon pulp, about 2 melons
Artificial sweetener to taste

Method
Purée pulp in a blender and strain. Mix well with milk, sweeten to taste, and freeze in an ice-cream maker. Serves 6. *23 calories per serving.*

Lemon Sherbet

Ingredients
3 lemons, grated and squeezed
1 cup water
Artificial sweetener to taste
1 egg white, beaten

Method
Add water to lemon juice and grated peel. Sweeten to taste, stirring until sweetener is dissolved. Let mixture rest for 5 hours. About an hour before serving, fold lemon mixture into beaten egg white and place in an ice-cream maker. Serves 6. *8 calories per serving.*

Presentation of sherbet: With soupspoons form ovals of sherbet and place two in the center of a flat plate. (Guérard would offer 2 flavors.) Surround sherbet with fruits arranged according to pleasing color combination: strawberries, raspberries, melon slices, mango slices, pear slices, cherries, apple slices—whatever is at hand. Serves 6.

DINNER
Artichoke à la Poule
Fish under Prairie Herbs with
Purée of Watercress
Lemon Pots de Crème

Artichokes à la Poule

Ingredients
½ pound mushrooms, diced
Salt and pepper
6 artichoke bottoms
6 poached eggs

Method
Sauté mushrooms in a Teflon pan. Purée them in a blender and season to taste with salt and pepper.

Poach artichoke bottoms in salted water for about 10 minutes. Drain. Spread each artichoke bottom with a layer of mushroom purée; nestle a neatly trimmed poached egg on top, and mask with a layer of mushroom purée. Serve at room temperature. Serves 6. *95 calories per serving.*

Trout or Sea Bass under Prairie Herbs with Purée of Watercress

Ingredients
3 branches wild mint
10 pieces clover, plus some for garnish
3 branches of nettles
2 fistfuls of meadow grass
2 fistfuls of hay
6 trout, about 6 ounces each, or
1 sea bass, about 2½ pounds, cleaned, but do not bone or
  scale
Salt and pepper
About 1 cup water

Method

In a deep oval iron casserole make a bed of half the herbs and grasses, lay the trout or sea bass on top, salt and pepper to taste, and cover with a blanket of remaining grasses. Add water; cover. If using trout, steam 5 minutes over very high heat; if sea bass is used, steam 15-20 minutes. Trout are served whole; sea bass is skinned and filleted. Sprinkle a few clover leaves on each fish. Reserve fish stock. *135 calories per serving.*

Sauce for Trout or Sea Bass

Ingredients

1 large carrot, julienned
½ cup mushrooms, julienned, plus 5 cut into quarters
About 4 tablespoons leeks, julienned
1 tablespoon celery, julienned
Salt and pepper
2 cups reserved fish stock
3⅓ tablespoons skim milk
1 tablespoon no-fat white cheese

Method

In a covered casserole, cook, without liquid, carrots, ½ cup mushrooms, leeks, and celery, seasoned to taste with salt and pepper, for about 8 minutes. Add fish stock and cook an additional 5 minutes. Drain and reserve stock.

In a saucepan cook quartered mushrooms in milk for about 7–8 minutes. Purée in blender with cheese and stock from vegetables.

Remove mixture from blender, add drained vegetables, mix well. Top trout or sea bass with sauce. Serves 6. *15 calories per serving.*

Purée of Watercress

Ingredients
4 bunches watercress
Salted water

Method
Cook watercress in salted water. Drain. Purée in blender.
Serve with fish. *13 calories per serving.*

Lemon Pots de Crème

Ingredients
7 tablespoons skim milk powder
2 cups hot water
Zest of 3 lemons
Artificial sweetener to taste
2 eggs beaten
Mint

Method
Preheat oven to 150°. Mix milk with water and delicately
stir in the zest and sweetener, beating constantly. Strain. Add
eggs and pour into 6 individual molds. Set into a pan of
water and bake for about 1 hour. Chill. Serve with sprigs of
mint. Serves 6. *40 calories per serving.*

LUNCH
Eggplant Caviar
Cider Poached Chicken
with Apricots
Orange à l'Orange

Eggplant Caviar

Ingredients
3 eggplants, about ½ pound each

Oil
½ cup mushrooms, diced very small
1 shallot, minced
1 small egg yolk
2 tablespoons fat-free white cheese
¼ cup tomato, peeled, cut into chunks, and diced
2 tablespoons red pimiento (tinned), diced
1 garlic clove, minced or pressed
2 tablespoons chervil
Juice of ½ lemon
Salt and pepper

Method

Preheat oven to 200°. Wash eggplants but do not dry. Remove caps and stems and slice stems in half lengthwise; blanch and set aside. Place eggplant on a rack, cover with a thin film of oil and cook for 20 minutes, turning occasionally. Slice eggplants lengthwise, remove flesh, leaving skin intact, and chop fine.

Sauté mushrooms and shallot in a Teflon pan and set aside.

In a mixing bowl, whisk together egg yolk and cheese and add eggplant and continue to beat until mixture is supple. Add tomato, pimiento, garlic, mushrooms, chervil, lemon juice, salt and pepper to taste. Pile mixture into eggplant shells, place on a plate, refit blanched eggplant stems. Chill. Serves 6. *71 calories per serving.*

Cider Poached Chicken with Apricots

Ingredients for vegetable farce
⅓ cup carrots, diced very fine
⅓ cup turnips, diced very fine
6 ounces veal, all fat removed and diced small
3½ tablespoons breadcrumbs soaked in 6⅔ tablespoons milk
2 tablespoons tomato, peeled, seeded, and chopped
2 eggs plus 2 egg whites
Handful of chopped parsley, chervil, and tarragon

Method for vegetable farce

In a bowl, mix all ingredients together. Fold a kitchen towel in half horizontally and along the folded edge spoon a line of the farce and roll the towel, shaping the farce into a sausage form. Tie the two ends tightly with string.

Ingredients for poaching chicken
1 2½ pound chicken
8 cups dry apple cider
2¼ cups young carrots, cut into olive shape
2¼ cups young turnips, cut into olive shape
2 cups zucchini, cut into olive shape
3 cups leeks, cut crosswise
Small cabbage, stem cut off and leaves removed
6 apricots

Method for poaching chicken

In a large covered casserole poach the chicken in cider with the carrots, turnips, zucchini, leeks, cabbage, and roll of vegetable farce in towel for 30 minutes. During the last 10 minutes of cooking, add the apricots.

Ingredients for applesauce
1 cup cider liquid
1 cooking apple, peeled, cored, and quartered
Grated peel of 1 lemon

Method for applesauce

At the same time you are poaching the chicken add cider, apple, and lemon peel to a saucepan and cook for 6–8 minutes. Sieve the apple or purée it in a blender, without the liquid; strain liquid and add about ¾ cup of purée.

Ingredients for assembling dish
Applesauce
Chicken cut into 6 serving pieces, skinned
Vegetables from poaching liquid

Vegetable farce cut into thick slices
Apricots, peeled, halved, stoned

Method for assembling dish

Spread each plate with a layer of applesauce, center a piece of chicken, and surround it with the vegetables from the poaching liquid, disposing them according to color. Place a slice of vegetable farce on each piece of chicken. Lay an apricot half on each side of the vegetable farce. Serves 6. *416 calories per serving.*

Orange à l'Orange

Ingredients

6 small oranges, peeled, and peel sliced into a fine julienne
Water
Artificial sweetener to taste
1 cup strawberries, puréed
1 kiwi or 1 kumquat, sliced lengthwise into 6 thin slices

Method

Place peel in a saucepan, cover with water, and add sweetener. Cook orange peel gently until it boils and continue 2 minutes.

Remove the white inner skin from the peeled oranges and carefully separate the sections.

On individual plates, spread a layer of strawberry purée, top with a layer of orange sections placed in a circle, like pinwheel petals of a flower, and at the heart place a slice of kiwi or kumquat. Sprinkle with orange peel. Serves 6. *69 calories per serving.*

DINNER
Asparagus Soufflé
Grilled Fillet of Beef
Chocolate Granité

Asparagus Soufflé

Ingredients
1 pound asparagus plus 18 stalks, woody ends removed and sides peeled
Salt and pepper
Pinch of mace or nutmeg
6 egg whites, beaten until firm
2 egg yolks

Method
Poach asparagus in salted water and drain well. Reserve 18 stalks and purée the rest in the blender. Season purée with salt, pepper, and a pinch of mace or nutmeg. Mix egg whites with purée and add yolks. Pour soufflé into six 4-inch individual molds and bake in 220° oven for 7–8 minutes. Cut points from reserved asparagus stalks and slice lengthwise. Before serving, decorate each soufflé with 3 asparagus points, halved. Serves 6. *60 calories per serving.*

Grilled Fillet of Beef

Ingredients
Water
6 juniper berries, crushed
1 branch thyme
¼ bay leaf, crumbled
6 fillet or beef steaks (about ¼ pound per person)
Salt and pepper to taste
3½ tablespoons parsley, chopped
3¼ tablespoons chervil, chopped
¾ teaspoons garlic, minced
2 shallots, minced
Juice of 1 lemon
3 leeks, cut crosswise into 4 sections
3 cups chicken consommé

Method

Mix water, berries, thyme, bay leaf, and dip steaks into mixture until just barely covered; this will keep them from sticking to grill. Grill on each side 2½ minutes. Salt and pepper steaks to taste.

In a bowl, mix parsley, chervil, garlic, shallots, and lemon juice, and spoon over top of steaks.

Poach leeks in 2 cups of consommé. Purée leeks in a blender, smooth consistency with about 1 cup consommé. Serve with steaks. Serves 6. *224 calories per serving.*

Chocolate Granité

Ingredients
2 cups water
1 vanilla bean
7 tablespoons skim milk powder
5 tablespoons cocoa powder
Artificial sweetener to taste
1 tablespoon heavy cream
1 cup frozen coffee crystals (recipe below)

Method

In a saucepan, combine water and vanilla bean and bring to a boil. Remove from heat, remove bean, and add milk, cocoa, and sweetener and stir well. Let mixture cool.

Add cream and mix well. Just before serving add mixture to an ice-cream machine and turn for 15 to 20 minutes; or place in a refrigerator tray and freeze for 1 hour. As liquid solidifies, turn with a fork a few times. At last moment stir in frozen coffee crystals. Serves 6. *32 calories per serving.*

Coffee Crystals

Ingredients
1 cup hot water
1 tablespoon decaffeinated coffee

Method

Mix ingredients, place in freezer, stirring with a fork a few times to form granulated crystals.

LUNCH
Tomato Tart
Blanquette of Veal with
Purée of Cauliflower
Coffee Pots de Crème

Tomato Tart

Ingredients

6⅔ cups tomatoes, peeled, seeded, and chopped, plus 1 tablespoon for garnish
1 shallot, minced
3 cloves garlic, minced
1 branch thyme
¼ bay leaf
Salt and pepper
4¼ pounds spinach, cooked and drained

Method

Preheat oven to 200°. In a saucepan, place tomatoes, shallot, garlic, thyme, bay leaf, salt, pepper, cook gently until liquid evaporates.

Line six 4-inch molds with spinach leaves, fill with tomato mixture, and cover with spinach leaves. Bake in oven for 15–20 minutes. Unmold and decorate with a bit of tomato. Serves 6. *128 calories per serving.*

Blanquette of Veal with Purée of Cauliflower

Ingredients

8 cups chicken consommé or bouillon
5 carrots, cut in large pieces
2 onions, cut in large pieces

1 leek, cut in large pieces
8 mushrooms, cut in large pieces
1¼ pounds veal from the leg, fat removed, and cut into
   chunks
Salt and pepper
Chopped parsley,
Peeled tomato
1 cauliflower cut into 4–5 pieces
Salted water

Method
   In a deep saucepan, add consommé or bouillon and
carrots, onions, leeks, and mushrooms. Wrap a kitchen towel
around a large strainer that just fits the pan, and place the
veal in the strainer. Cover and steam the meat over the
simmering liquid for about 45 minutes. The veal will be
faintly rose-colored at interior. Remove vegetables and whirl
in the blender. Season with salt and pepper. The vegetable
mixture serves as the sauce; if it is too thick, add a little of
the poaching liquid.
   Place veal on a platter and top each portion of veal with a
spoonful of sauce. Sprinkle with parsley and a bit of peeled
tomato. Cook cauliflower in salted water, drain, and purée in
a blender. Correct seasoning. Serves 6. *194 calories per
serving.*

Coffee Pots de Crème

Ingredients
7 tablespoons skim milk powder
2 cups hot water
2 rounded teaspoons decaffeinated coffee powder
Artificial sweetener to taste
2 eggs, beaten
Frozen coffee crystals (recipe on p. 278)

Method

Mix milk powder with water and delicately stir in the coffee and sweetener, beating constantly. Strain. Add eggs and pour into six individual custard cups. Set into a pan of water, bake in a 150° oven about 1 hour. Chill. Serve with a few sprinkles of coffee crystals. Serves 6. *40 calories per serving.*

DINNER

Carrot Kugelhupf with Chervil
and Purée of Artichoke
Brochettes of Scallops with
Sauce Sabayon
Melon with Strawberries

Carrot Kugelhupf with Chervil and Purée of Artichoke

Ingredients

2¼ cups carrots, sliced fine
4 tablespoons water
2 tablespoons butter
½ cup chicken consommé or 1 teaspoon powdered chicken
    consommé
Salt and pepper
10 tablespoons diced mushrooms
1 shallot, minced
2 eggs
2¼ tablespoons Gruyère, grated
1 rounded tablespoon chervil or parsley
Clarified butter

Method

In a large pot, cook carrots, water, butter, consommé cube or powder, salt and pepper to taste. Pass through the largest disk of a vegetable mill.

Sauté mushrooms in a Teflon pan with the shallots; a few turns in pan will suffice. Mix mushrooms into the carrot purée.

In a bowl, mix eggs, Gruyère, chervil or parsley, and combine with carrot purée.

Line the interior of a medium-sized, glazed terra-cotta mold (for kugelhupf) with a thin film of butter. Pour in the carrot mixture and set the mold in a pan of water. Cook in a 200°–220° oven for about 45 minutes. Serves 6. *99 calories per serving.*

Purée of Artichoke

Ingredients
3 artichoke bottoms, cut in quarters
3 asparagus tips
Salted water

Method
Poach artichoke bottoms and asparagus for about 10 minutes. Drain. Purée in a blender. Serves 6. *4 calories per serving.*

Note—Guérard presents the unmolded carrot kugelhupf on a chopping board strewn with green resinous leaves of a thuya tree, resembling a form of ferns.

Brochettes of Scallops with Sauce Sabayon

Ingredients for court bouillon
1 cup white wine
1 cup water
1 cup carrots, cut into eighths
½ cup leeks, cut into eighths
6 small onions, sliced
Branch of thyme
½ bay leaf
Salt and pepper
2 tablespoons fresh tarragon, chopped.

Method for court bouillon
In a saucepan, place wine, water, carrots, leeks, onions,

thyme, bay leaf, and season with salt and pepper. Simmer mixture for 15 minutes. Remove 15 tablespoons of court bouillon to another saucepan, add tarragon, reduce by half. Set aside.

Ingredients for brochettes
30 scallops
1 large tomato, cut in quarters and again in sixths
3 large mushrooms, quartered
1½ bay leaves

Method for brochettes
   Thread 6 metal skewers (which can be totally immersed in liquid) with 5 scallops each alternating with 4 tomato sections, mushrooms, and a spear of bay leaf at each end. From this point in the recipe one must move quickly.
   Bring court bouillon to a simmer and add skewers and cook for 4 minutes.

Ingredients for sauce sabayon
Reserved court bouillon with tarragon
2 tablespoons water
2 large egg yolks

Method for sauce sabayon
   Simmer the bouillon. In a bowl, whisk water and egg yolks to a froth, doubling its volume. Remove bouillon from stove and add egg/water mixture and whisk again. Pour sauce over brochettes and rush to the table. Serves 6. *97 calories per serving.*

Melon with Strawberries

Ingredients
3 cantaloupe melons, cut in half and seeded
1 cup strawberries

Method
    With a small melon scoop make a ring of indentations in each melon half. Fill center of melon and indentations with strawberries. Serves 6. *42 calories per serving.*

Lobster Ragout

Ingredients
1 2-pound lobster
Court bouillon (recipe on p. 282)
1 tablespoon olive oil
Cognac
White wine
Fresh tomato
Fish fumet°
Sauce à l'americaine °
Mushrooms
Sauce sabayon (recipe on p. 283)
Garnishes: glacéed small onions, carrots, turnips, and cucumbers

Method
    Remove claws from lobster and poach them in court bouillon. Detach the tail and cut the trunk in 2 parts. Remove coral, set aside.
    Cook the tail and trunk in a heavy enameled skillet in olive oil for about 10 minutes. Remove and set aside. Deglaze the skillet with cognac, white wine, fresh tomato, fish fumet, and sauce à l'americaine. Strain and set aside.
    In a blender purée mushrooms and coral. Add to sauce to give it more consistency and keep warm.
    Open the shell of the lobster tail with a pair of scissors, and cut meat into large pieces. Reconstruct half the lobster on each plate; in the shell of the body place the meat from the claw.

    ° Recipes can be found in standard French cookbooks or in *Larousse Gastronomique.*

Lighten the sauce with a small amount of sauce sabayon and spoon on the lobster. Garnish each plate with onions, carrots, turnips, and cucumbers. Serves 2.

Pigeon Salad

Note: A dark-fleshed game bird—quail, pheasant, guinea hen—is nearest substitute if pigeon is unavailable; but recipe could be adapted to Cornish hens or chicken.

Ingredients
1 pigeon
Pigeon consommé or chicken stock
2 or 3 leaves of 2 or 3 different salad greens like romaine, spinach, rugola, or a variety of lettuces
Vinaigrette sauce
12 artichoke bottoms, halved
1 tomato, peeled, seeded, chopped
1 tablespoon kernels of corn
1 tablespoon mushrooms, cut in strips
1 tablespoon lemon peel, cut in strips

Method
Remove legs from pigeon, and grill. Poach rest of pigeon in pigeon consommé (or well-flavored chicken stock) until cooked but still rose-colored. Slice thin. Dress greens with a light vinaigrette sauce. Arrange each plate with grilled thigh in center surrounded by greens on which are laid thin slices of poached pigeon. Ring with halved artichoke bottoms, sprinkle over remaining ingredients. Serves 2.

Chapter 31

WEIGHT, WISHFUL THINKING, AND WILLPOWER

• The U.S. Public Health Service reports that from 25 to 45 percent of the American population over thirty years of age is more than 20 percent overweight.
• In April of 1975, there were counted some 27,960 methods of weight loss on public record.
• A New York psychiatrist has invented a special mirror for his overweight patients that shows what they would look like thin.

WHAT NEXT?

Three recognized experts in the field of overweight and obesity research have come up with some answers—Dr. Marci Greenwood, Assistant Professor of Human Genetics and Development at the Institute of Human Nutrition, Columbia University; Dr. C. Peter Herman, Assistant Professor of Psychology at Toronto University, specializing in research on human consumption; and Dr. Dale G. Friend, Associate Clinical Professor of Medicine Emeritus, Harvard Medical School, and a practicing physician.

COUNTING FAT CELLS INSTEAD OF CALORIES

Probably many people know that obese people have up to

five times as many fat cells as normal people of the same age and height, but according to Dr. Marci Greenwood, there are *two* kinds of obesity, one which involves a higher fat cell *number*, and the other which involves a higher fat cell *size*. "Weight reduction," she explains, "whether in adult or child, reduces fat cell *size* only. Therefore, hypercellular obese people (i.e., with too *many* fat cells) even when reduced to normal weight have too many, too small fat cells." So you can be thin, but it's harder work to stay that way because you have more fat cells to nourish.

The other fact stressed by Dr. Greenwood concerns children. "In normal animals and presumably in humans as well, fat cell number is 'set' early in life. Obese children may develop as many fat cells by two to five years of age as are found in normal *adults*." She urges that more attention be paid to the nutrition of the very smallest babies in order to prevent the number of fat cells from multiplying in an abnormal fashion. Much of Dr. Greenwood's work now focuses on the question of whether we can stop this development of fat cells, and also "whether we can learn to accept a certain degree of overweight in some individuals (who have a large number of fat cells) as perhaps unfortunate for them but nonetheless *normal for them*."

OVERWEIGHT OR UNDERFED?

Dr. C. Peter Herman agrees with Dr. Greenwood that it is possible, if you are endowed with a large number of fat cells, to be overweight by societal norms but *under*weight by biological norms. In fact, he points out, "There is a remarkable similarity between obese humans and starving humans. Both show greater emotional reactivity and greater distractibility. Eating behavior is similar. The extent of the parallel is sufficient to suggest what many overweight people have been saying for years: They're starving!

"Finally," Dr. Herman adds, "I do not intend to convey

that the fact that you have an excessive number of fat cells will doom you to a life of obesity or even overweight. It may doom you to a life of having to worry about your weight. If people couldn't diet successfully—even in the face of clamoring fat cells—they wouldn't be biologically underweight, would they? So the moral of the story is that weight loss is possible."

THE FRIENDLY WAY

Dr. Dale G. Friend, who sees many overweight patients in his practice, makes a plea for more sympathy and support for these people. "The terrible burden borne by the obese, which makes them maladjusted to the society around them, is one that needs more understanding and compassion," he says. "A determined effort by parents, physicians, public health agencies, and society in general should be made to prevent obesity developing in the child and to help those already afflicted to overcome it by encouragement—emotional, physical and psychological."

Dr. Friend's special knowledge is in the field of drugs. "Crash diets, unbalanced diets, various drug regimens, hypnosis, and many other temporary programs are all to be condemned, as they do not get at the fundamental problem and lead to a yo-yo type of recurrent obesity. They do more harm than good." Dr. Friend also mentions that there is a strong hereditary aspect to obesity. "If both parents are obese, there is about a 70 percent chance that children will be obese. If one parent is obese, there is a 30 percent chance of obesity developing in the child."

Dr. Friend, as a practicing M.D., says that he cannot claim a higher than 30 percent recovery rate for his overweight patients—roughly the same as for drug or alcohol addiction. So how does he treat the problem of overweight?

"First and most important, you must remember it is a long, even lifetime business. You can only begin with that in mind."

Four guidelines for weight loss from Dr. Friend
1. Get at the psychological problem. Review your life and try to get the emotional things straightened out.

2. Do not take in excess energy over what you can burn. This means cutting down your intake of calories. There's no short-cut to this. Miracle diets will not help—they may lose you a few pounds, but then they come right back again.

3. Find a doctor or nutritionist who has enough interest in you and pays enough attention to you to keep you coming back, facing the scales, and talking over your problems. Then any patient will respond and do what is necessary—it's a two-way street. (If you cannot find a doctor who will give you this help, some hospitals have nutritionists in their out-patient clinics who can advise you.)

4. For your children's sake, practice preventive medicine. Stop believing, like your grandmothers, that a fat baby is a healthy baby, or that sweet cereals and sodas are normal foods for children. Give them the minimum of sweets, however much they like them. They'll thank you in the end.

The Peril of Pills

Dr. Friend has a special word to say about placebos. "The workings of the human mind are very strange—if we believe a thing strongly enough, it becomes true. For example, acupuncture works exceedingly well in China where they believe that it works. But there are plenty of papers coming out in the U.S. just now on the minimal effect of acupuncture here—because the people do not believe in it. If a person has a firm belief in a placebo, say an appetite reducer, then it may work for a while. But in the end, it will wear off and you are back where you started. Even with medically effective drugs this happens (amphetamines, for instance, do suppress appetite). The patient becomes 'tolerant'; for instance, you may get tired of taking the drug; you may build up enzymes in your body which destroy the efficacy of the drug; or your body simply does not react any more.

"In other words," says Dr. Friend, "if you are going to lick the fundamental physiological defect, you have to get right down to the fundamental principles—your emotional state, your outlook on life, your personal habits—and reeducate yourself insofar as food, energy intake, and expenditure are concerned."

Dr. Friend also has some encouragement to offer. "There are some strong-willed people who can lose weight on their own," he says, "but most of the human race do not have that kind of will power. We have it for a while, but it has to be reinforced. Do not expect too much. *Find someone to help, listen, check your scales and diet, follow your progress with interest.* That way, you will keep trying, and find it possible to succeed."

One more encouraging thought: Dr. Greenwood mentions that the people of a certain African tribe have a unique distribution of fat on their bodies regarded within the tribe as highly desirable. This phenomenon is presumed to have come about through cultural influences. It is possible, she therefore speculates, that if we continue to believe that fewer fat cells are beautiful, perhaps in several generations hence we may be born that way—an example of how cultural adaptation could help us all become slim—naturally!

Chapter 32

HOW TO GEAR YOUR MIND TO THINK YOURSELF SLIM

Do you think that the only way to lose weight is to go on a diet? Do you think that failing at weight control means there's something wrong with you? Do you hate what you see in the mirror? If you say "yes" to all these questions, you are probably one of the millions of Americans who have tried to lose weight with the hundreds of weight-loss techniques on the market today; and you are also probably one of the millions saying, "It's no good, I just can't keep it off. I give up."

Well, take heart. Help is at hand from a group of psychologists—a not-surprising quarter, considering the dramatic trend toward mind-and-body medicine that is beginning to influence the health profession. Dr. Frances Meritt Stern, Associate Professor of Psychology at Kean College, and Director of the Institute for Behavioral Awareness in Springfield, New Jersey, explains the breakthrough: "I once asked a large group of women to raise their hands if they thought restrictive dieting was the way to lose weight. The great majority raised their hands. Then I asked them, 'How many of you are now normal-weighted because of restrictive dieting?' Ninety percent of the hands went down. *Yet they didn't see the connection.*

"We work in cause-and-effect logic: which means we help you develop the kind of control where you are pulling the strings on yourself. We help you help yourself—and that's how you learn self-control."

Dr. Stern's approach is "thought restructuring." The idea is that your mind is some sort of computer, programmed a certain way, with negative, erroneous thoughts about yourself, your food, your relations with other people, and the world. Dr. Stern's colleagues help you to reprogram your mind with more positive, assertive, appropriate statements.

This is actually an example of behavorial therapy, but at the Institute for Behavioral Awareness, the techniques are specifically geared to overweight people with their particular attitudes and feelings. The mind exercises that Dr. Stern has developed for these people are highly original and demonstrably effective, and with her program coordinator, Ruth S. Hoch, she has collected many of them in a book entitled *Mind Trips to Help You Lose Weight* (Playboy Press, $8.95). (Both Dr. Stern and Mrs. Hoch lost weight dramatically by this process: In one year, Dr. Stern lost 48 pounds and Ruth Hoch over 60 pounds—and they have both kept it off.)

"We've taken the behavorial method and applied it to the general human condition," explains Dr. Stern. "When people first come to us, we ask them to fill out an interview sheet that asks questions such as, 'What's important in your life?' 'What do you think your biggest success is?' 'What do you say to yourself when you overeat?' We want to show people that if they've been successful failures, they can also be successful successes. Most people can help themselves, but they simply don't know how." The ultimate goal of this process is to liberate yourself from the vicious cycle of being upset, overeating, and becoming more upset. Here are seven exercises developed by Stern and her colleagues that may help you change your mind to change your weight:

1. List 20 things that turn you on. Many people learned to overeat because food was given as a reward—you've been a good girl, here's a cookie. Dr. Stern suggests that you list 20 everyday things that are pleasurable, and begin to use them instead of food as rewards. "They do not have to be something you buy or do. They can be 'mind trips.'" For instance, Ruth Hoch imagines seeing her two children, who are both away—and that makes her feel good. It can be that simple.

2. Ten-finger exercises. "We recommend you learn this," says Stern. "*You can eat two tablespoons of anything and not get fat.* Not everything, but anything. Now for that to sink in, try saying it ten times, once on each finger, 'I can eat two tablespoons of anything I like.' That way, you program it into your mind. Another ten-finger exercise is to say to yourself, 'I have an unconditional right as a human being to be happy.' For some people, only by repeating that idea ten times a day can they begin to believe it. Eventually, what you have programmed in by this exercise becomes part of your thinking and will come to mind whenever you need it."

3. Eat what you shouldn't eat. People often say they simply cannot stop overeating. "Fine," says Dr. Stern, "Let's make sure you *really* can't stop. Set a timer, and every ten minutes, you have to eat—for an eight-hour period. If you have a certain passion for, say chocolate doughnuts, then eat one every day. You'll find that you can stop all right. I had a client who compulsively ate chocolate doughnuts, and after making her eat one a day for some time, she finally came to me and said, 'I'm ready to quit.' And I said, 'No, you're not.' You must go past the point where you don't want the food any more. The point is not that she began to hate them but that she was *allowed* to have them. Before, they were forbidden fruit, and that was the compulsive factor."

4. What you say to yourself when you binge eat. Binge eaters usually talk to themselves while they eat, and what they say is very negative. "I hate myself." "Why am I doing this?" "Is something wrong with me?" They torture themselves while they eat. Dr. Stern asks that you question these negative statements. "Are you capable in any other ways? Is there anything else you have done besides eat? Do you run a household? Look after children? Work hard at your job?" Dr.

Stern tries to replace the punishing thoughts with positive ones, so that the binge eater can cope better and become more creative when faced with food. In this context she also suggests you develop a side-tracking technique, such as imagining a place where you have been happy or feel comfortable, and bring it to mind clearly, with sounds, smells, colors, and so forth: This helps you enjoy pleasant feelings without recourse to food.

5. Rehearsing. "There are many times when you want to control your eating, but can't bring yourself to do it," says Dr. Stern. "But you can do it in your head. That gives you internal practice. Say you're going to a wedding, where there will be wall-to-wall hors d'oeuvres. Try rehearsing going into the room, seeing the food, and acting appropriately. This gives you an idea about how you can control yourself, how you can be in charge. We simply teach you that you are responsible. Then when the real-life situation happens, you are prepared and can cope with it."

6. Analyze what you want to eat. "When you eat, try and get involved in your food. Notice the taste, savor it on your tongue, start enjoying it," suggests Dr. Stern. "Then, when you begin to feel like eating something, analyze precisely what taste it is you want. Overweight people tend to crave food—to eat for the sake of eating—and as they do not know what they really want, they are never satisfied. Try to select out what you are after in terms of taste, and then go for that, nothing else. This will prevent you from consuming a lot of junk food that won't satisfy you." Dr. Stern tells clients if it's sweetness they really want, "take a teaspoon of sugar. It's eighteen calories of pure sweetness, much better for you than devouring twenty cupcakes."

7. Partner support. Dr. Stern's treatment involves the clients' spouses or partners, if they have them. "We ask them to catch their wives or husbands doing something *good*," she says.. "It's easy to catch them snacking. But it's much more helpful to reinforce their good behavior." Sometimes the husband or wife of the overweight person becomes threatened by the possible change in the personality of the spouse through the loss of weight. Dr. Stern's colleague, Ruth Hoch, recalls the situation where the husband always used to bring home cake for his wife, who was in the weight-control program. "The truth was, he did not want her to change. But as often as he brought the cake home, she would throw it out, and finally he stopped and accepted the fact." Dr. Stern explains that this is a well-known syndrome, and should be understood by husband and wife. "Some people choose to remain overweight," she says. "What they are getting from being overweight is more valuable than getting thin. Maybe losing weight would put too much stress on the marriage."

Most couples, however, in Dr. Stern's experience, can benefit enormously from the weight-control program. "As a person loses weight, he or she becomes a more positive, confident person, and this carries over into the marriage. Someone who feels good about him or herself will be a better person to live with. And to have support from your partner while undergoing weight loss can have a value that is much more profound than the simple encouragement—it can bring out a new strength in the relationship, and a new confidence both individually and with each other."

These are just some of the techniques that are used at the Institute for Behavioral Awareness. You will notice that going on a restrictive diet is not one of them. "It's hard for people to accept this idea," says Dr. Stern. "Yet it's what's going on in your mind that affects your body, and what we are doing is getting at your mind, at all the wrong thinking that makes you overeat. Failing at weight control doesn't mean anything is wrong with you, or that you are a wicked person. It simply means that you are not using your mental skills properly, or that you do not have those skills in your repertoire, and must learn them." By changing your attitude to a more positive approach, you can liberate yourself from guilt and learn to cope with everything in life more successfully.

How much do you really know about weight control?

Dr. Stern has come up with 5 important questions about weight
that show whether you understand the underlying truth
about losing it. Test how much you know by marking the boxes
—not what you think is right, but what
you really *feel*—then look below for the answers.

1. Losing weight requires a great deal of willpower.

True ☐ False ☐

2. Many people seem naturally to overeat.

True ☐ False ☐

3. Food seems to jump into your mouth.

True ☐ False ☐

4. Some people don't have the ability to imagine.

True ☐ False ☐

5. Your mind and your body are separate parts of yourself.

True ☐ False ☐

ANSWERS TO WEIGHT CONTROL QUIZ

1. False. "Losing weight requires self-control, not will
power," says Dr. Stern. "Will power is a negative concept—
in the sense of avoidance, it simply doesn't work. Not
everyone has will power. People without will power, for
instance, may have to spill water over their food or flush it
down the toilet, so as not to eat it. But you can learn to lose
weight without will power. Self-control can be learned, step
by step, without involving will power."

2. False. "You *learned* to overeat," Dr. Stern says, "and you learned it well. But if it's learned, it can be unlearned, and more appropriate responses substituted."

3. False. "This is what we mean by self-control. *You* are responsible for what you eat—not 'it'—not the food."

4. False. "Do you sometimes worry? What is happening then? You are using your imagination in a negative way. We suggest you use the same skill in a positive way. You have the skill—it needs developing, to help you lose weight."

5. False. "How you feel about yourself and what you say to yourself affects the way you eat. That's why we must attack the way you feel about yourself, and change that, rather than change the food by putting you on a diet. That is also why diets so often fail. We have to change your *mind* to change your weight."

Chapter 33

LOW-CALORIE ENTERTAINING WITH HEALTH IN MIND

American cook and author Helen Corbitt has been creating food to lose weight by for years, as food consultant to The Greenhouse Spa in Texas. She is often asked for party food that's tempting, delicious, yet light and low in calories. Here are her ideas for four menus that will delight guests and keep you healthy; plus some low-calorie hors d'oeuvres.

Menu 1:
Crabmeat Chantilly
Cold fresh asparagus and avocado with capers and crisp, diced bacon, lemon juice, and oil dressing
Rye melba toast
Cold poached whole peaches with burnt-sugar threads

Low-Calorie Crabmeat Chantilly

Ingredients
1 tablespoon whipped margarine
1 tablespoon shallots, minced
1½ pounds crabmeat, fresh or canned, or any cooked seafood
¼ cup dry white wine
5 egg whites
2 teaspoons cornstarch
1 tablespoon Dijon mustard

1 teaspoon salt
Few drops Tabasco sauce
¼ cup Parmesan cheese, grated

Method

In a large saucepan melt margarine, add shallots, and sauté for 1 minute. Add the crabmeat and stir with a fork. Add the wine and simmer until the wine has evaporated. Pour crabmeat into a light greased 1½-quart casserole.

In a bowl beat egg whites until soft peaks form. Add the cornstarch. Continue beating until the whites are stiff. Stir in mustard, salt, and Tabasco. Cover the crabmeat mixture with the egg white mixture and sprinkle with Parmesan cheese.

Place in a 350° oven until hot and lightly brown on top (about 20 minutes). Serves 8. *101 calories per serving.*

Note: A light cream sauce may be substituted for the wine and shallots, without increasing the calorie count. And you can also make a richer mixture by substituting 1 cup mayonnaise for the cornstarch.

Menu 2:

Demitasse of cold squash soup with raw asparagus spear to stir
Boiled brisket of beef with natural juices
Spinach and green pea soufflé
Steamed fresh cabbage chunks sprinkled with finely chopped pine nuts
Celery salad with mustard dressing
Compote of fresh steamed pears, apples, and plums in red wine and cinnamon

Cold Squash Soup

Ingredients

1½ cups onions, finely chopped
2 tablespoons whipped margarine
1 quart summer squash, sliced

2 cups chicken broth
Pinch of sugar substitute (optional)
2 cups skim milk
Salt
White pepper
Parsley or chives, chopped

Method

In a saucepan add onions to margarine and sauté over low heat until soft and yellow.

Add the squash and broth. Cook until the squash is tender. Add the optional sugar substitute. Let the squash cool, then purée in a blender.

When cold, add milk and salt and pepper. Refrigerate. Serve with asparagus spears to stir with. Serves 6. *12 calories per demitasse serving.*

Spinach and Green Pea Soufflé

Ingredients

1 tablespoon whipped margarine
1 tablespoon shallots or onion, finely chopped
3 tablespoons flour
1 cup skim milk
4 egg yolks, beaten
1 cup fresh spinach leaves, washed, dried, finely chopped
1 cup fresh or frozen peas, cooked, drained, mashed
5 egg whites, stiffly beaten
⅛ teaspoon salt
White pepper

Method

In a large saucepan melt the margarine, add shallots, and cook 1 minute over high heat.

Add flour and cook until foamy. Add milk and cook, stirring, until thick. Cool slightly.

Beat in egg yolks and add spinach and peas. Fold in the egg whites, salt and pepper.

Pour into a lightly oiled 2-quart soufflé dish, and bake at 375° for about 40 minutes. Serves 10. *70 calories a serving.*

Menu 3:

Cottage or farmer's cheese soufflé

Sautéed sherried mushrooms

Pineapple shell filled with apricot sherbet, surrounded with fresh pineapple fingers and fresh mint

Cottage Cheese Soufflé

Ingredients

4 eggs, separated

Pinch of salt

1 teaspoon flour

¼ teaspoon dry mustard

Pinch of cayenne

1 cup sour cream

6 ounces dry cottage cheese, softened at room temperature, or 6 ounces of farmer's cheese (if cream cheese, calorie count goes up to 210 per serving)

Method

In a large bowl beat egg yolks until thick and creamy. Add salt, flour, mustard, and cayenne.

In another bowl combine sour cream and cheese; blend until smooth. Add to egg yolks; beat until smooth.

In a bowl beat egg whites until stiff but not dry and fold into yolk mixture. Put mixture in an ungreased 1½-quart soufflé dish.

Place in a pan of hot water and bake in a preheated 300° oven for 1 hour. Serves 6. *95 calories per serving.*

Apricot Sherbet

Ingredients
4 cups apricot nectar, hot
1 cup water-packed apricots, chopped finely
1 3-ounce package lemon gelatin
Juice 1 lemon
Artificial sweetener, if necessary
Ice
Rock salt

Method
In a bowl mix nectar, apricots, gelatin, and lemon juice together and freeze in an ice-cream freezer with 6 parts of ice to 1 part rock salt.

Or freeze in a deep freeze and whip when partially frozen in an electric mixer and return to freezer. Makes 1½ quarts. *45 calories per ½-cup serving.*

Menu 4:
Pâtés of lobster and breast of chicken with a light sweet-and-sour sauce.
Artichoke soufflé ring filled with julienne carrots with vodka and grated orange peel
Fresh lime milk sherbet in fresh coconut shells

Pâtés of Lobster and Breast of Chicken

Ingredients
2 8–10 ounce lobster tails deshelled and cut into 1-inch pieces
2 8-ounce chicken breasts, skinned, and cut into 1-inch pieces
1 cup sherry
½ cup butter, melted
Salt
White pepper

Method

Thread lobster and chicken alternately into 6 buttered or oiled skewers. (I use bamboo and throw away after.) Place in a shallow pan, pour wine over and refrigerate until ready to cook. Drain, season with salt and pepper.

Bake at 350° for 10 minutes, then under the broiler for about 5 minutes. Baste with the wine and butter.

Correct seasonings; serve either on the skewer or slip off but retain shape. Serves 8. *170 calories per serving.*

Sweet-and-Sour Sauce

Ingredients
1 cup pineapple juice
¼ cup vinegar
1 teaspoon arrowroot

Method

Mix juice, vinegar, and arrowroot together and stir until smooth and thick. Heat until smooth and clear. Makes 1¼ cups. *7 calories per tablespoon.*

Artichoke Soufflé Ring

Ingredients
2 tablespoons whipped margarine
2 tablespoons flour
½ cup skim milk
1 teaspoon onion, grated
Salt, white pepper
4 egg yolks, beaten
2 cups canned artichoke bottoms, mashed (broccoli may be used)
5 egg whites, beaten stiff

Method

In a large saucepan melt margarine; add flour; cook until bubbly. Stirring with a whisk, add milk, and cook until thick.

Add onion and season with salt and pepper. Add egg yolks and artichokes. Let mixture get cold. Fold in egg whites.

Pour into a lightly greased ring mold. Set in pan of hot water. Bake at 350° for 45 minutes. Let stand 10 minutes, unmold.

Fill center with julienne carrots or snipped green beans. Serves 8. *90 calories per serving.*

Julienne Carrots

Ingredients
6 medium, fresh carrots, washed, scraped, and cut in julienne
    strips
¼ cup vodka
Grated zest of 1 orange
Salt, white pepper

Method
In a casserole sprinkled with Pam or vegetable oil, add carrots and vodka, and cover.

Bake in 350° oven for 25 minutes. Season with orange zest, salt, and white pepper. Serves 6 to 8. *50 calories per serving.*

Low-calorie Hors d'Oeuvres

Small raw mushrooms filled with mashed Roquefort and
    cottage cheese
Celery brushes filled with mashed marinated fresh salmon
    and caviar
One-inch cucumber boats filled with diced tomatoes, celery,
    and capers
Cherry tomatoes split and filled with tiny shrimp
Small tomatoes scooped out and filled with cheese soufflé
Jacima scooped out, filled with Jacima fingers
Jellied poached eggs with truffles
Tomato baskets filled with tiny shrimp

CELEBRATE—AND STAY SLIM

Teas and tisanes—infusions of herbs and dried wild-flowers—are wonderfully restorative to body and spirits, and usually zero in calories. Sip a cup while preparing seasonal culinary treats. Or serve an herbed tea or tisane as an invigorating meal starter.

Elegant Bubbly

Delightful to the eye and palate and a winner in the slimdown race

Ingredients
2 bottles (a fifth each) California sauterne, chilled
2 bottles brut champagne, chilled
1 orange, thinly sliced, then halved
1 lemon, thinly sliced, then halved

Method
Float a block of ice in a punch bowl and add the sauterne, then the champagne. Add the slices of orange and lemon. Serve in flute or tulip champagne glasses. Add an orange or lemon slice half to each glass. Serves 24.

Yerba Maté

An unusual tea—Yerba Maté—is especially appropriate at Christmas, as it's made from dried holly leaves. The plant grows wild in Paraguay, Brazil, and Argentina, and is extremely popular in South America. Brew the maté as you would tea. Add lemon or a few cloves, cinnamon, or allspice for interesting flavor. Maté is available at herb and spice and health shops.

Tisane Americaine

Michel Guérard serves his own tisane, a concoction of herbs, pine needles, heather flowers, and the like, at his famous spa at Eugénie-les-Bains, as an apéritif. Here is a stateside version made with native herbs.

Ingredients
3 teaspoons dried clover blossoms
2 teaspoons marigold flowers
1 teaspoon lemon balm
¼ teaspoon borage
3 cups water, brought to a boil
Lemon slices

Method
Place herbs in teapot, pour boiling water over them, and let the tea steep 5 minutes, Strain and pour into small mugs or teacups and serve with a slice of lemon.

The tea may be chilled and served in juice glasses, a slice of lemon to each.

Bits of fruit—apple, pineapple, orange, grapefruit—may be added after steeping. Serves 4.

Molly's Pitcher
Fruity and kicky

Ingredients
1 cup (1 9-ounce can) pineapple tidbits, drained, but reserve 2 tablespoons of the pineapple liquid.
2 fresh tangerines, peeled, white membrane removed, and segmented
12 ounces blended rye whiskey
6 ounces peach brandy
14 ounces 7-Up
Fresh mint leaves

Method
In an old-fashioned, quart-sized pottery or pewter pitcher,

put drained pineapple tidbits, pineapple liquid, and tangerine. Add whiskey and brandy. Stir and let stand at room temperature 1–2 hours to macerate.

When ready to serve, add ice cubes and 7-Up. Stir and pour into pewter mugs, with a few pieces of pineapple to each. Top with a sprig of mint. Serves 6 to 8.

Tea à la Casablanca

Minty, invigorating—*exotic*

Ingredients
8 teaspoons green tea or 8 teabags
⅛ pound spearmint leaves, dried
1 quart water, brought to the boil
½ cup sugar or equivalent sugar substitute

Method
Place tea and spearmint leaves in a large teapot or pitcher. Pour boiling water over the leaves and steep 3 to 5 minutes. Add sugar or sugar substitute if desired. Strain into porcelain teacups and serve at once. Serves 6.

Variation on a Mimosa Theme

Pretty bubbly—and very much à la mode

Ingredients
Block of ice
1 quart orange juice, chilled
1 large grapefruit, peeled, seeded, and cut into small segments
2 or 3 oranges, peeled, seeded, and segmented
1 magnum sparkling white wine (such as Kriter or Blanc de Blancs), chilled
1 quart carbonated water

Method

Float a block of ice in a large punch bowl. Add the orange juice and fruit segments.

Add the sparkling white wine and carbonated water. Serve at once in coupe champagne glasses with a piece or two of segmented fruit in each. Serves 24.

Delicious Golden Punch

Refreshingly tangy—and rewardingly low in the calorie department

Ingredients
1 cinnamon stick, about 2 inches long
20 whole cloves
1 quart cold water
10 teaspoons of leaf tea or 10 teabags
1 quart apple cider
2 cups cranberry cocktail juice
Juice of 1 lemon
Raw cranberries, to garnish

Method

Add cinnamon stick and cloves to water and bring to the boil. Take off heat.

Place tea leaves or bags in a large pitcher and pour in spiced water. Steep tea until a deep amber color. Strain into a large punch bowl and cool.

When ready to serve, float a block of ice in the spiced-tea punch bowl and add remaining ingredients. Serve in stemmed all-purpose wine glasses. Add 3 raw cranberries to each glass. Serves 16–20.

Hot and Spicy Cider

May be prepared several days in advance, a definite advantage at the holiday season

Ingredients

2 quarts sweet cider

4 3-inch sticks of cinnamon

1 tablespoon whole cloves

1 teaspoon ground ginger

½ teaspoon allspice or 10 cloves

6 pieces or orange zest, about 3 inches by ¼-inch wide, plus more for garnish

Method

Place cider, spices, and orange zest in large pot and bring to the boil. Lower flame at once, simmer, covered, 30 minutes. Cool.

Strain and pour into covered container. Refrigerate overnight, or 2 to 3 days.

When ready to serve, heat to the boiling point and serve piping hot in ceramic mugs. Add a curl of fresh orange zest to each mug. Serves 20 to 24.

TIPS FOR MIXING LOW-CALORIE DRINKS

A squeeze of lime, the juice of a grapefruit, a spicy broth, plus a liberal jangling of ice cubes all add a fillip and the minimum of calories to a drink. Here are some snappy tips for low-calorie mixing, great new recipes for light drinks, and a calorie chart for spirited drinks.

Know your calories

The caloric content of distilled spirits may be calculated entirely on the basis of alcohol content.

DISTILLED SPIRITS	
Gin, rum, vodka, whiskey	
80 proof	
Jigger (*1½ fluid ounces*)	**97**
1 fluid ounce	**65**

DISTILLED SPIRITS		calories
86 proof		
Jigger / 1 fluid ounce		105 / 70
90 proof		
Jigger / 1 fluid ounce		110 / 74
94 proof		
Jigger / 1 fluid ounce		116 / 77
100 proof		
Jigger / 1 fluid ounce		124 / 83
CARBONATED WATERS		
Sweetened (quinine, tonic) / 1 fluid ounce		12
Unsweetened (club soda)		0

Think melon

Fresh melon has many things going for it—zingy flavor, low calorie count, pleasing texture, terrific eye appeal. Puréed or liquefied, it is frothy, cooling, pastel-colored, and makes a superb base for many mixed drinks. One half cup of cubed cantaloupe, enough for 1 drink, is 24 calories; casaba melon, 31; honeydew, 27; watermelon, 21.

Here are some *Minceur Melon Mixers* using techniques of the slimming new-wave cooking of France. Use them as ideas; mix and match your own melon mixers.

Honeydew and Rum Minceur: Combine ½ cup cubed fresh honeydew, 1 ounce rum, and whirl in a blender or food processor until puréed. Spoon into an Old-fashioned glass, add plenty of crushed ice, and stir. Garnish with a cube of fresh cantaloupe. Calorie count: 97.

Cantaloupe and Vodka Minceur: Combine ½ cup cubed fresh cantaloupe, 1 ounce vodka, and 1 teaspoon fresh lemon juice in a blender or food processor and whirl until puréed or liquefied. Spoon into a double Old-fashioned glass; add ice cubes and a splash or two of club soda. Calorie count: 92.

Casaba and Brandy Minceur: Combine ½ cup cubed fresh casaba melon, 1 ounce brandy, and 1 teaspoon lemon juice in a blender or food processor and whirl until liquefied. Spoon into a tall glass, add plenty of crushed ice and a splash or two of club soda. Calorie count: 100.

Watermelon and Gin Minceur: Place 1 cup seeded and cubed watermelon and 1 ounce gin in the blender or food processor and whirl until liquefied. Pour into a tall glass, add plenty of ice cubes, and 3 slightly bruised juniper berries. Calorie count: 89.

The Slim Americano: Mix 1 ounce Campari, 1 ounce sweet vermouth, and a dash or so grenadine extract, which has a pomegranate flavor. Add lots of ice, plenty of club soda, and garnish with a twist of lemon zest. Calorie count: 110.

Orange Mountain Fizz: The zesty fruitiness of California Mountain Red Burgundy marries tastefully with the flavor of orange. The addition of Curaçao reinforces the flavors and provides an automatic intensity.

Use a tall slim Collins glass. Add 2 ounces California Mountain Red Burgundy, ½ ounce Curaçao (or other orange-flavored liqueur), and lots of crushed ice. Fill glass with diet orange soda. Top with 1 large beautiful Emperor grape. Calorie count: wine, 46 calories; Curaçao, 48; total, 94.

Jamaica Jolt: Three flavors enliven each other and make a refreshing drink, attractive to the eye, palate, and waistline.

Chill a balloon wineglass. Fill it ⅓ full with crushed ice. Add 6 ounces freshly brewed and cooled strong tea, and strained juice of ½ freshly squeezed lime, and 1 ounce light rum, 80 proof. Stir and garnish with a sprig of dark, leafy Italian parsley. Calorie count: lime juice, 7 calories; rum, 67; total 74.

White on White: Here's a spirited white on white that's high in taste. The herbs in the vermouth are not apparent to the eye, but they give the drink a pleasant zing.

Chill an old-fashioned glass. Pour in 2 ounces dry Italian vermouth, 3 ounces dry white California Chablis or Chardonnay, and add enough ice cubes to fill to the brim. Stir. Garnish with a sprig of rosemary. Calorie count: vermouth, 70; wine, 43; total, 113.

Sherry Apple Spritzer: The delightfully nutty flavor of the amber sherry lingers long on the palate. The apple juice gives a buoyance to the sherry, and the club soda turns the whole into a spritzer. Note: Dry cocktail sherry or fino sherry usually contains many fewer calories than do the heavier oloroso and cream sherries.

Pour 2 ounces dry cocktail or fino sherry, 3 ounces unsweetened apple juice into a stemmed tulip wineglass. Add crushed or cracked ice and a splash or so of club soda. Stir well and garnish the drink with a thin, unpeeled slice of apple. Calorie count: sherry, 75 calories; apple juice, 30; total 105.

Sake Icecap: The Japanese traditionally drink Sake warm, in tiny porcelain cups, but in recent years it's become fashionable to drink Sake on the rocks, Western style. Its piquant flavor is surprisingly refreshing and gentle in a tall, cold drink and blends well with green tea, which is known as "the white wine of teas" in Japan.

Fill a tall, thin glass ⅓ full with crushed or cracked ice. Add 3 ounces Sake and fill with green tea that has been prepared with tea leaves, then cooled. Stir and garnish with a thin slice of lime. Calorie count: Sake, 75; total, 75.

Quick tips for reducing calories in mixed drinks

Lemon—A teaspoon of lemon juice, fresh or bottled, adds zip and tartness to tomato and fruit-based drinks and contains only 1 calorie.

Lime—Gimlet and Lime Rickey lovers will be delighted that 1 teaspoon of fresh or bottled unsweetened lime juice adds just 1 calorie to the drink.

Unsweetened Grapefruit Juice—Fresh or frozen, unsweetened grapefruit juice adds up to 12 calories per ounce.

Bouillon or Beef Broth—A fantastic mixer, invigorating and satisfying; both marry well with whiskey. Commercial bouillon cubes contain as little as 6 calories per cube, 4 ounces of canned beef broth as little as 6 calories. (Campbell's prepared beef broth, 4 ounces, 13 calories; College Inn, 6 calories.)

Clam Juice or Liquor—For those who love the taste of the sea, clam juice is fresh, bracing. Four ounces are 16 calories.

Tomato Juice and Vegetable juice cocktails—6 ounces of zingy tomato or vegetable juice cocktail contain from 31 to 43 calories, depending on the brand. (V-8 is 31; Campbell's tomato juice, 33; College Inn tomato juice cocktail, 43.)

Drink Garnishes—Stay with a curl of lemon or orange zest, or a thin slice of fresh lemon or orange, and little cocktail onions, which contain only trace calories.

Water—Nature's perfect noncaloric mixer, lengthens every drink without adding to the calorie count.

Ice Cubes and Crushed Ice—The festive clink of ice, like a conditioned reflex, adds to the pleasure of a drink and the gaiety of the occasion.

Crushed Ice turns a standard cocktail into a frappe, which not only looks pretty, but lasts longer.

Club Soda—The sparkling effervescence gives a tingle to the tongue and extends a modest amount of whiskey or wine into a lingeringly long drink.

Diet Sodas—Especially for those who like their drinks on the sweet side. These will add only trace calories to any mixed drink.

Part Four

EXERCISE: THE HEALTHY BODY IN ACTION

Today, exercise is as much a part of life as eating and sleeping. There are many different ways of exercising—you can do it yourself, as an independent activity, or you can participate with others in all the various sports available. Whatever you choose, if you do it right, your body will feel the difference—for the rest of your life.

Chapter 34

EXERCISE ROUND-UP

"Whenever I feel the urge to exercise, I lie down until it passes." The late Robert Hutchins, President of the Center for the Study of Democratic Institutions, is credited with that remark. *Newsweek* columnist George F. Will broadly defined exercise to include "vigorously pushing away from the table and strenuously snuffing out cigarettes."

The wretched fact is that even though we know we should exercise (and nearly one half of the Americans who do exercise do it for reasons of health), the idea somehow doesn't fill us with wild enthusiasm. We can understand the concept of exercise meaning *play*—for instance, tennis, swimming, or any activity we define as "sport"—but when health gets into it, the fun seems to go out of it.

"The way we live is our number-one health problem," declares V. L. Nicholson, spokesman for the President's Council on Physical Fitness and Sports. "This is the first major change in our health attitude since the forties. In earlier days, infections such as TB and diphtheria were still major killers—now it is our own bad habits. People simply must begin to see how important exercise is in keeping them in shape."

The President's Council is deeply involved in trying to get the youth of America to start the exercise habit. "The growing years are vital," says Mr. Nicholson. "What children do between the ages of ten and fifteen affects the size of their heart, lungs, the quality of their bones, everything. So youngsters should get systematic activity." He observes with regret that this is more difficult to achieve with girls than with boys. The National Youth Fitness Test turns up the unfortunate truth that whereas before puberty boys and girls usually develop their strength, speed, stamina, and agility at the same rate, at puberty girls level off or stop completely. They've reached their peak. "Maybe it has a little to do with physiology, but not all. I'm afraid it's also sociological," admits Mr. Nicholson. "For some reason, girls feel that physical activity is no longer worth doing—a mistake that they may pay for dearly in later life."

Well, we're *trying.* More Americans are exercising now than ever before and, probably owing partly to the Women's Movement, more women are involved in sports than ever before. The tennis boom has swept the country. More and more people are building swimming pools for exercise—and more of them are indoors so the exercise can go on all year. You see joggers on every street in every town—there is even a National Jogging Association based in Washington, D.C. (In 1972, a National Adult Physical Fitness Survey found that of the 60 million adult Americans who engage in various forms of exercise, nearly 44 million walk for exercise; more than 18 million ride bicycles; 14 million swim; 14 million do calisthenics; and 6.5 million jog. The survey did not even bother to include tennis as a category that year.)

The latest excitement in exercise, and one that is sweeping California is the fitness *parcours.* The word *parcours* is French for "course," and the idea originates from Switzerland, where the fitness *parcours* is very popular. The *parcours* is a walking-jogging course with 20 exercise stations along the way, where you rest from jogging, and do various stretching, bending, and other fitness exercises before moving on to the next one. Deborah Mazzanti has a fitness *parcours* at her health spa, Rancho La Puerta, and believes it is the exercise trend of the future. "Anyone can do it," she says, "and it's fun. The *parcours* is portable: It would be perfect in parks, for the whole community to enjoy, or even in your backyard if it's big enough."

It is not just health nuts who are becoming exercise-minded. There is a whole new class of American exercisers—older people with cardiovascular disease. "Heart attack patients used to have to stay in bed," Mr. Nicholson says. "But now there are highly sophisticated exercise techniques for such patients, based on heart rate and oxygen delivery systems, which help them lead normal active lives again. This is another major change in our attitude to health in the past thirty years."

There is still enormous resistance to exercise. People say it's boring, they haven't time, they don't need it. In 1972, 49 million Americans never exercised at all (that's nearly half the adult population). But let's face it, we do need it. Here are some ways of working out that four famous exercise specialists recommend and that may surprise you because you'll feel so terrific afterwards. So terrific that if you keep it up for three months, you'll be hooked. As Deborah Mazzanti put it, "A daily exercise routine makes the difference between *existing* and *living*."

Indoor Exercises

"If the weather is so bad that you can't venture outdoors, jump rope," says Dr. Lenore R. Zohman, Director of Cardio-pulmonary Rehabilitation, Montefiore Hospital, and member of the Exercise Committee of the American Heart Association. "Jog in place or, if you have one, ride a home bicycle. You should also choose activities that put all your joints through their entire range of motion. For instance, bicycle riding does not exercise your arms, so you should do some arm exercises in addition. Ideally, you should do some form of calisthenics to use all the joints and stretch the muscles, plus some form of endurance exercise to raise the heart rate—but to a target level, 220 minus your age for most healthy people. Puffing and panting like a sprinter is not necessarily helping your heart and maybe just tires you out."

Bicycling

"The muscles that suffer most in winter are the leg and abdominal muscles," says Dr. Willibald Nagler, Chief of Physical Medicine and Rehabilitation, New York Hospital, "so I recommend bicycle riding, which is very good for the legs. You should really ride for about an hour to get any benefit, and since you do not use your arms, do some arm exercises as well." As for the abdominal muscles, here is a very good exercise from Dr. Nagler: Lie on your back, bend your knees. Do a half sit-up, hold it for 5 seconds, then let down. "This is also very good for people with back problems, incidentally," he says. "If you have access to an indoor pool, swimming in my view is still the best overall exercise there is."

Skating

People tend to think of skating as something beautiful to watch, but it's also wonderful exercise, according to Dr. Tenley E. Albright, of Sports Medicine Resource in Woburn, Massachusetts. (Dr. Albright won the Olympic Gold Medal for Figure Skating in 1956, so she should know!) "Any kind of movement, anything which increases agility, including climbing on the rocks by the beach in summer, prepares you for winter skating. Before you start, take a good look at your skating boots and make sure they fit snugly around the ankle, loosely at the toe and the top of the boot. I'm sure you'll find, as I do, that skating is not just great exercise, it's something you'll look forward to doing!"

Jogging

"Jogging is excellent exercise," says Dr. Nagler, "as long as you are in good physical condition. Jogging on snow is all right, but people who jog constantly on concrete can come up with joint problems, so watch where you do it. Also, in winter, you should start slowly, because your air tubes or lungs can contract in very cold weather when the cold air reaches them." The effect is rather the same as when you put your fingers in the freezer for any length of time. Cold air imposes an added load in the system, so if you have bronchial trouble, consult your doctor before setting off on a jogging program. "Otherwise, my advice is, build up slowly— a thirty-minute jog is perfectly adequate for most people."

Cross-Country Skiing

"Cross-country skiing is phenomenal exercise," says Dr. John L. Marshall, Director of Sports Medicine at New York's Hospital for Special Surgery, and orthopedist for the U.S. Ski Team. "It is mainly an endurance sport and it has the same effect as jogging, playing tennis, or swimming—activities you can't do so easily in winter. But remember this vital rule: *You should get in shape to play rather than play to get in shape.* This means you should have some knowledge of the sport first before you try it, and also good strong legs and abdominal muscles—which means sit-ups." Dr. Marshall feels the key to winter sports is flexibility, so warm up to some degree before you start—especially important for people over thirty-five. Cross-country skiing—and its companion, downhill skiing—are tremendous exercises but make great demands on the body. "One of the members of the New York Giants football team once came to see me complaining of stiffness after skiing—right at the end of the football season when he was in peak shape! So for those of us who aren't Giants, be even more prepared."

BASIC PROGRAM FOR ALL SHAPERS-UP

The President's Council on Physical Fitness and Sports recommends the following routine, whatever form of exercise you decide to practice:

1. 7–8 minutes of warm-up. Stretch, bend, twist, turn, generally loosen up, and breathe a little harder.

2. 8–10 minutes of strength work on arms, shoulders, thighs, etc., with push-ups, sit-ups, pull-ups.

3. 20 minutes of circulatory exercise at a pace that elevates breathing and heart rate. *Not* all-out effort, just a regular pace. Jogging, fast walking, bicycling, running, skipping rope—any brisk activity will do for this period.

4. 5–7 minutes of cool-down. Don't sit down abruptly after finishing your exercise, but move around slowly staying loose for a while before resting.

MOREHOUSE ON MORE FITNESS

Dr. Laurence E. Morehouse is one of the foremost authorities in the field of fitness. It was his physical fitness program that enabled the astronauts to work successfully on the surface of the moon, and it was a machine invented by him that NASA adapted to keep the astronauts fit while they orbited the earth. He is Founding Director of the Human Performance Laboratory at the University of California, and author of several books on fitness.

"Fit for what?" demands Morehouse as he watches out of his laboratory window business executives huffing and puffing at their miles of jogging. "Why should you take on an exercise program that's geared to a long-distance runner if you're not going to run a marathon? Fitness strictly relates to your ability to meet the demands of your environment—and my program hits at the key elements to change for the *average* person, not the athlete—it *does no more and no less than you need to do.*

"Man is meant to be an active animal. When he's not active, he falls apart. Joints become stiff; you begin to get aches and pains—signs that changes are taking place. The back is a good signal that things aren't right—most of us have back problems. Another sign is feeling out-of-breath after climbing stairs. All definite signs your body is not getting the activity it needs to maintain good physical condition.

"It is the rigidity in exercise programs that in my opinion is the reason people are turned off to exercise. 'I just can't do it,' people say. 'I just can't keep it up, so why bother to do it at all?' It's not human. My approach is, let's be human about exercise. Do it till it feels good and till you don't want to do it any more and then stop—and it's okay. If today is my day to exercise and I don't feel like exercising, say I'm tired or off-key a little, no big deal. I won't exercise today, and tomorrow maybe I'll feel better. If you miss a couple of days, it's okay. Routine is good as long as it's not compulsory—because if you can't keep up the routine, then you tend to feel like throwing out the whole program. If you *want* to exercise every day because it satisfies you or relieves your guilt feelings, then that's fine, too. But my exercise program is designed to stop anyone feeling guilty about exercise ever again!

"You don't have to buy equipment. But if it makes it easier for you, then have it. Mrs. Morehouse has a stationary bicycle.

"You can start at any age—I studied eighty-year-olds who were practically bedridden, and after a careful program of exercise, checking their pulse, they've come back to good condition—playing tennis, even. You can change your fitness in a month from poor to good. Fitness is temporary. You lose about five percent every three days if you don't exercise. That is why it's best not to skip exercise more than two days in a row."

Dr. Morehouse's program of exercise is based on your pulse rate. However it beats at rest, it's your pulse rate during exercise that enables you to structure your fitness program exactly to your requirements. (The only people for whom this does not apply are those whose doctors have forbidden exertion or who have special pulse-rate problems.) Your resting pulse while seated averages about 72–76 beats for men, and 75–80 for women. In general, the lower the resting heart rate, the more efficient you are. You need to get your pulse up for a few minutes a day to maintain a healthy heart. Once you are in fairly good condition, you will avoid physical deterioration if you meet 5 requirements every day, says Dr. Morehouse.

1. Get your heart rate up to 120 beats a minute for at least 3 minutes.

2. Turn and twist your body joints to their near-maximum range of motion.

3. Stand for a total of 2 hours a day.

4. Lift something unusually heavy for 5 seconds.

5. Burn up 300 calories a day in physical activity.

This is simple. And so are the exercises that Dr. Morehouse has devised—and demonstrates at the end of the chapter, to make you fit and healthy without guilt in 10 minutes a day, 3 times a week.

Start with 4 limbering exercises. Use whatever rhythm pleases you. Don't count—there's no need. Just spend about 15 seconds on each exercise.

Once you are stretched and limbered, you are ready to develop muscle tissue. Expansion sitbacks—to restore muscle of the abdominal wall—and expansion pushaways should be done twice each for a total of about 4 minutes, alternating them as you feel inclined. As you become more fit, increase difficulty of pushaways by lowering hands below shoulder height, as he does himself. The remaining 5 minutes of your exercise program are for good circulatory conditioning. The "Endurance Lope" will raise your heart rate to your proper level for 5 minutes.

More Fitness Tips

If you do these exercises for 10 minutes a day, 3 times a week, says Dr. Morehouse, you will have good muscles, good circulation, and an improved cardiovascular system. For people who want to maintain fitness for sports and athletic activities, these exercises can be stepped up. It's up to you. Your pulse will tell you how much effort you're expending. And the exercises are so simple to do, unlike some of the exercises we have all been led to believe are so wonderful, such as touching your toes, deep knee bends—all of which, declares Dr. Morehouse, do more harm than good.

Keep Cool! "Sweating weakens you," declares Dr. Morehouse. "Always exercise with light-colored, light clothing, not sweat suits or warm-up suits. In my program with the astronauts we experimented to see what happened if we allowed their body heat to rise. We found that just a slight increase in temperature markedly decreased the person's capacity for physical work."

Look for Fitness Opportunities. "During the day, don't lie down when you can sit. Don't sit when you can stand. Don't stand when you can move. When you wake up, have a good stretch. When you wash, soap and dry yourself vigorously. When you walk, walk briskly. And look for opportunities to *climb stairs.*

"I've had people who can't stand exercise—any kind of exercise. But one thing they will do is climb the stairs once in a while. This will improve their condition markedly. Now older people tend to buy houses all on one floor in order to avoid stairs. 'I'm past fifty,' they say. 'I don't want stairs to climb any more.' *The opposite is true*—the older you get, the more you need those stairs. This doesn't mean you have to run up and down them all day. But people looking for retirement homes should look for stairs. It may be all the exercise they are going to get.

"A cardiologist is looking for two things," explains Dr. Albert A. Kattus, former Chairman of the Exercise Committee, American Heart Association, and Professor of Medicine (division of cardiology), University of California at Los Angeles. "One, exercises that are safe for people with heart disease to do; and two, ways to encourage people to adopt habits of activity that may forestall the possibility of heart disease. To my mind, walking is the ideal exercise for both situations."

Greta Garbo's walks are her religion. When Lilli Palmer once collected her off Onassis's giant yacht, she complained, "It is too small! I cannot go for my walks!" Rose Kennedy still walks 3 or 4 miles a day. Here, four special walking experts give their prescriptions for getting the most out of walking, and show why becoming a walker could be the best thing you ever did for the rest of your life.

1. HOW A WALK CAN KEEP YOUR HEART HEALTHY

"The beauty of walking is that it is measurable," says cardiologist Dr. Kattus. "You can measure a mile, and how long it takes to walk it. For heart patients, this is vital. We do a multistage walking test on a treadmill to establish how much exercise people with heart disease can take without risk, and then start them on a walking program taking into account the work load he or she can tolerate—gradually increasing it over time. The trouble with bicycling is that it is too easy on the level, and too hard on uphill, for heart patients. Jogging and running are also totally different kinds of exercise that require skill, training, and experience.

"For a normal healthy person, with no symptoms of heart trouble, the 4-mile-per-hour walking test is quite easy. But the problem with many people is that they do not walk nearly enough in their daily lives. At Los Angeles airport, there are even mobile sidewalks, so you do not have to walk at all! We recommend that normal people who lead relatively sedentary lives should walk regularly each day, as fast as possible, for anything from 20 minutes to an hour. The fastest most people can walk is 4½ miles per hour, and that is not making a high demand. But 2 or 3 miles like that every day will counteract the dangers of a sedentary life.

"If you have no time to walk that much, or nowhere to walk, then try walking upstairs instead. Anything to keep moving! Remember that walking uses up calories, too. Here are some examples, taking a person who walks 3½ miles per hour—a good, brisk walking pace: 1 hamburger (350 calories) takes 60 minutes to walk off; 1 glass of beer (113 calories) takes 22 minutes; 1 large apple (100 calories) takes 19 minutes; 1 fried egg (110 calories) takes 21 minutes; 1 malted milk shake (502 calories) takes 95 minutes! And remember, if you *don't* walk, these calories will simply pile up. Incorporate walking into your daily life. Your heart will reap the benefit."

2. HOW TO PUT YOUR BEST FOOT FORWARD

"The ideal way to walk is on the outer borders of your feet with your feet pointing straight ahead," explains podiatrist Dr. Roberts. "You should put the weight first on the heel, then along the *outer* border of the foot and then across the toes, ending with the big one. Your shoe will often tell you if you are walking correctly. If the outer border of the heel and the *inner* border of the sole are worn down, that's wrong. It should be the outer border that is worn, all the way round.

"For walking, wear the lowest heel you can comfortably wear. For women used to wearing high heels all their lives, a very low heel may not be comfortable. Open toes will be more comfortable for many women than closed toes, particularly if you throw your weight forward a lot. Open toes and open heels are often the easiest to walk in, if you are not walking over rough terrain.

"Do not worry about ankle support. Podiatrists have long

since learned that the stability of the ankle is the result of the stability of the foot. Sprained ankles are often due to a person not walking properly. Big shoes and boots are necessary mainly for protection against hard country.

"Choose leather or fabric that allows your feet to breathe and is flexible. Plastics, patent leathers, and reptile are difficult to wear and tire the foot as they have no 'give.' Soles should be leather or ripple or crepe rubber as long as they are flexible.

"Sneakers are very good for walking as long as there is some cushioning in the heel against hard walking surfaces. But if you need arch support, do not expect to get it in the arch raise built into sneakers. Arch supports must be placed in a shoe according to the individual need. Negative heel shoes (where the heel is lower than the sole) have certain advantages—space for toes, a wide shank, snug heel, lightness, and flexibility. But people who are not accustomed to walking in them will find them very tiring, because of the pull on the leg muscles. Manufacturers now recommend that customers wear the shoes for just a few hours every day to get used to them." (Dr. Nathaniel Gould, former Chief Orthopedic Surgeon at Brockton Hospital, Massachusetts, and former President of the American Orthopedic Foot Society, Inc., has done extensive tests on these shoes with his colleagues, and they have concluded that they are twice as tiring as sneakers in the long run. The effect is as though you are constantly walking uphill. But some feet may all the same find them very satisfactory—it's a personal matter.)

"Wear cotton or wool socks," advises Dr. Roberts. "There should be something between you and the shoe. Following these guidelines, your feet should enjoy the walk as much as you do. If you get very tired walking, probably something is wrong with your feet. If this is a problem, consult a podiatrist in case you have a particular foot characteristic that should be compensated for in your shoes."

Tips on buying good walking shoes
1. Buy your shoes with the understanding that, provided you keep the shoes clean, you can get your money back if they are not comfortable. ("Any responsible shoe store will agree to this," says Dr. Roberts.) Take the shoes home; put them on; cover them with a shoe bag or big socks and walk about in them indoors for a couple of hours. That's the only good way to test their comfort.

2. Tests for a well-fitting shoe: (a) The heel should fit snugly. (b) The toe should be ¼ inch longer than your longest toe. (c) The shank—middle of the shoe—should be wide enough so your foot is not hanging over it at either side. (d) The front of the shoe should be broad enough so you can ripple the leather over the toes with your fingers. This is a better test than wiggling your toes, which you can do in almost any shoe. (e) Stand in the shoe on one foot—this is when most weight is expended onto the foot.

3. THE LASTING JOYS OF WALKING

"You don't have to have fields or wild flowers or parks to enjoy walking," says Mrs. Ruth Goode, author and passionate walker. "Walking on city streets has its own special joy. You become sensitive to where it is comfortable to walk according to the weather. For instance, I find that the East Side of New York City is cooler than the West Side in the morning and the reverse is true in the afternoon. If there's a wind blowing, it may be colder and windier on the West Side. You learn where the sun hits and where it is in shadow. Walking downtown in the wintertime along Central Park West is a delight—the sun is full on you, while the East Side is bleak and in shadow. You discover all these things as the seasons change.

"The best walking tip I can think of is: *Lengthen your stride.* Everything seems to fall into place then. All those tight back muscles let go; shoulders drop; neck loosens; head comes up; and that top-heavy upper body leans at just the right angle to make each step almost automatic without effort. And it all happens when you let your legs swing from the hip to take the longer stride. Hard-pressed executive types, both sexes, should particularly take note of this. I've seen men dutifully walk home from their offices, clutching their attaché cases full of work still to be done—but they walk so stiffly and tensely that one wonders if the walk is doing them any good. If they would only lengthen the stride—begin by measuring steps according to the cracks in the pavement—it really works.

"It's what you're doing in your head also that's so great in walking. You're shedding other things, making a transition from where you've come from to where you're going to be. Walking gives you time to get there in your head. That's invaluable, because we're assaulted with so many things we have to do, that we want to do, that we undertake to do, and with so much irrelevant sensory input in our daily lives, we have to block out things as we go. Walking does that for you.

"Freedom of motion is essential while walking. Wear nothing tight around you. Layer your clothes—a T-shirt and sweaters, varying in weight, so as you get warmer or cooler you can take things off or put them on, remembering that they should be light, as you have to carry them. Choose cushiony soles if walking in the city. Some people like walking sticks—or pick one up en route if they are going for a country walk—the rhythm of walking with a stick is very pleasant.

"There are lots of ways of walking. Some people have to have a purpose or destination, such as looking at birds or picking berries. Others walk just for the walk's sake. Some people won't walk unless they have company. Others will only walk alone. It depends on your own personality and what kind of walking you did when you were growing up.

"Children often don't see the point of walking, but if you show them, it's something they will value all their lives. I think we make delightful habits out of things we enjoyed as children. Interest them in walking by showing them the wild flowers and identifying them, or by hunting for berries and picking them."

4. HOW TO WALK FARTHER THAN YOU THOUGHT YOU COULD

(Aaron Sussman is coauthor of *The Magic of Walking*. He is a professional photographer, so he walks a lot, particularly in the country. He came up with this technique to help a friend, stranded during a city transit strike.)

"Remember Tom Sawyer painting the fence? You don't paint a whole fence, you paint a little bit at a time. If you are going on a walk and feel you can't make such a long distance as the one planned, interrupt your consciousness of distance by focusing on something else. Concentrate on conversation or your train of thought. This way you simply forget that you are walking such a distance. Nor do you get tired because you aren't aware you are supposed to be getting tired.

"Another tip is to try to walk as the Indians do—keep your feet parallel and quite close together, with your hands positioned so that the thumbs can brush your thighs as your arms swing."

Chapter 36

RUNNING—THE NEW HIGH

Q. What's the difference between running and jogging?
A. Runners go faster than joggers, take longer steps, and hence extend the knee more. There are more joggers than runners.

"I sleep much better."
"My energy's way up."
"My temper's improved."
"I'm much more relaxed."
"I've never felt better in my life."
Who are these lucky people and why are they in such wonderful shape? They're *runners*. They don't walk or skip; they run, several miles a day, and it's changed their lives.

Running used to be something you did to catch a bus, or watched in breathless admiration on Olympic tracks. Now it is becoming an activity as addictive as all those nasty habits we want to give up—only this habit is healthful, exciting, and psychologically therapeutic, and it's sweeping the country.

"Runners will tell you that the effect starts after they've been running a few minutes, and it persists for many hours after they have run," explains New York endocrinologist Edward Colt, physician for the New York Marathon, participant in metabolic studies projects on runners, and a runner himself. "They feel much calmer; they sleep better; and they're able to handle day-to-day problems more easily."

You only have to look at dogs, Dr. Colt points out, to see the effects of running. After your dog has had a good run, he becomes calm and well-behaved for the rest of the day. "Clearly there is some kind of physiological effect. We don't know yet precisely what it is. It is the subject of a lot of investigation by psychiatrists and physiologists."

We all know that we feel better when we exercise, and that if we don't exercise, we pay the penalty, but runners seem to experience more than just a normal physical sensation of satisfaction. Dr. Colt says he has met a large number of runners who have given up alcohol, coffee, and cigarettes since they started running. Your state of mind really seems to change. Runners quite literally become addicted to running, and feel distressed if they cannot run every day. Indeed, Dr. Richard O. Schuster, podiatrist and running specialist, suggests that running might be used as a treatment for addicts such as alcoholics or drug users. "Running has the same effect as drugs," he says. "You get a high and don't want to stop. Maybe it would be possible to get people to transfer their fix from drugs to running."

Nobody yet quite knows why running causes this state of euphoria, but when pressed, Dr. Colt speculated that it might affect the distribution of fluid in the body. "It seems that large alterations in fluid distribution in and around body cells affect your mood. Running may regulate these movements of fluid."

Well, speculative or not, more and more Americans are discovering that running is better than chamomile tea for calming the nerves. City parks and country lanes are increasingly filled with enthusiastic runners. Magazines such as *Running World* and *Running Times* tell you how to run and where the latest marathons are being held. Women's running in particular is gaining popularity. The New York Academy of Science's recent conference on the marathon concluded that women can and should run long distances, and that a women's marathon event should be included in future Olympic games. And a book exclusively on running for women has now been published, *Running for Health and Beauty*, by Kathryn Lance (Bobbs-Merrill).

Nonrunners tend to think running means getting out of breath and feeling exhausted after 2 minutes. Not so, says Dr. Colt.

"The recommended way is to run at a speed that lets you carry on a conversation. Most authorities feel that if you're out of breath, you're running too fast." In other words, running isn't really hard physical exercise at all. "I think most long distance runners will tell you that *hard* running is the one thing to avoid. They try to run smoothly and never stress themselves unduly."

The key to running, according to Dr. Colt, is to start very slowly, a few minutes every day, and build up a routine gradually. "Don't make the mistake of doing too much too soon. You may find it boring at first, but that's only a reflection of your poor tolerance to this new stress. As soon as you build up physical tolerance, the feeling of pleasure and exhilaration starts."

As for the nuts and bolts of running. Dr. Colt's advice is to wear *good running shoes* with arch supports and the maximum amount of sole cushioning (see "A Running Start" at the end of the chapter). "If your shoes are uncomfortable, it may mean you are going to have bruises, tendinitis, or other problems." Beginners should start running on as soft a surface as possible, such as grass or sandy ground, rather than on the road, which can be hard on ankles, knees, and even hips. (The foreign editor of *The New York Times* recently took up early-morning running in sneakers on the city streets. Not long after, he tore a calf muscle playing tennis, and was out of action for 6 weeks. His doctor attributed the injury to his running on cement in the wrong shoes. So be careful!)

Running on city streets raises another problem—air pollution. To run, you have to inhale and exhale more frequently than normal. How important, therefore, is the quality of air for a runner? The precise answer is not known, according to Dr. Colt, but even if the air is polluted, it is probably better to run than not take any exercise at all. Running cleans out the sinuses, lungs, and air passages generally. Dr. Colt recommended running to one patient who had intractable headaches from chronic sinusitis, which disappeared, never to return, when the patient became a regular runner.

Dr. Colt himself runs 5 miles a day; when he is in training, the mileage can increase to 10 a day. He usually runs in the evening, in the park, where he meets fellow runners. "As a group they are very relaxed and easy to get on with. We have great conversations as we run," he says. Those body fluids again. And if you've ever wondered what runners think about as they pound away, studies have shown that "élite" marathon runners think about running and nothing else. They concentrate on their style, on their breathing, on the way their feet are hitting the ground. Average runners, on the other hand, seem to indulge in a lot of daydreaming, fantasy, and thinking about their problems, "sometimes forgetting them too," adds Dr. Colt.

Running is one of the few athletic activities in this highly competitive society that is not competitive—which makes its new popularity particularly interesting. "Most runners find eventually that running is actually more important than competing," comments Dr. Colt. "Although some may compete, what the majority runs for is the feeling of well-being." Isn't that what we're all chasing after? On with your running shoes, America.

FINAL WARNING: Running really may be addictive. Runners often find they cannot get through the day without running. Are you prepared for that?

THE BIOMECHANICS OF RUNNING

If you thought professional runners just put on their running shoes and started to race down the track, you're in for a surprise. Podiatrist Dr. Richard O. Schuster, Professor of Biomechanics at the New York College of Podiatric Medicine, runs a highly specialized laboratory in New York devoted to *orthotics,* i.e., the science of standing, walking, and running. "The biomechanics of running is the engineering of running," Dr. Schuster explains. "If a person develops persistent pain, it is usually due to structural imbalance, and what we do in our work is to try and identify these imbalances and correct them with shoe inserts." Dr. Schuster points out that runners have special problems, particularly impact problems. "For instance, when you run, the force that occurs when your feet hit the ground is sometimes 2 to 3 times body weight. Because of the pounding process in running, if there is an abnormal motion in the foot, these extra forces will cause a problem."

The most common imbalance is developmental, meaning the soles of the feet tend not to be parallel to the ground, but instead the outer edge of the foot is lower than the medial (inner) part. (As Dr. Schuster points out, before we're born we're wrapped up into a ball; much of our growing up involved straightening ourselves out of that little bundle.) This means each time the foot strikes the ground during running, the ankle and arch drop medially. As a result the complaints most often heard from runners are ankle and arch pains. Carefully tailored arch supports can prevent the drop of the arch and excessive play on the ankle joint, often completely relieving such pains. Biomechanical imbalances can develop from even minor abnormalities of the structure of the feet and legs, which can lead to pain in any part of the leg, including knees and hips. Fortunately, some of these can now be corrected by suitable orthotics.

Looking at the amazing inserts Dr. Schuster makes in his laboratory, one might feel that to start running in regular sneakers is rather naive. But, Dr. Schuster is reassuring. "If you want to run a mile 3 times a week, then biomechanical imbalances are not much of a concern. If you can perform your daily living and working routines without any physical problem, then running 5 miles a week should be no problem either. After all, your body has learned to adapt to your biomechanical structure ever since you grew up. Only when people run as much as 30 miles a week can basic imbalances start to cause trouble. And today we are almost able to predict who will have problems and who will not, because we can estimate an individual's degrees of imbalance. A wealth of information is coming out of our biomechanical research."

Dr. Schuster does, however, suggest certain guidelines when choosing running shoes:

1. They should have thick soles, and thicker heels. The whole base of the shoe should be filled in. These shoes help reduce the possibility of Achilles tendinitis, and are available at most shoe or sporting-goods stores.

2. They should have a flexible sole where the major joint is, under the ball of the foot, rather than under the arch, where most shoes flex.

One other piece of advice from Dr. Schuster: Don't run when in pain. "A runner or jogger should work on the premise that pain is damaging." If you feel pain while running or afterwards, consult a doctor.

A RUNNING START

1. Wear arch-supported sole-cushioned running shoes (see Dr. Schuster's advice above).

2. Run just a few minutes at first and build up slowly. Run on a soft surface if you can.

3. Run at a speed that lets you carry on a conversation.

4. If you have had heart or chest trouble, consult your doctor, and be particularly careful. If you feel that you are out of breath, you are stressing yourself excessively.

5. Don't eat a big meal before you run.

Chapter 37

DANCING—THE FUN EXERCISE

One of America's favorite movie moments was when Yul Brynner, as the dignified, undemonstrative King of Siam, finally "got down" and danced with Deborah Kerr. "And perchance," he sang, "when the last little star has leaved [sic] the sky/Shall we still be together with our arms around each other . . . shall we dance? Shall we dance? Shall we dance?" The polka, as dances go, is not exactly a great emotional liberator. But the King of Siam was charging, galloping, really cutting loose. Dance (just about any kind) does that to a person (just about any person). "It's so therapeutic," says Zita Allen, who writes about dance and has been studying it since she was eight years old. "I feel complete control over my whole body, a fantastic sense that I can get my body to do what it's supposed to do. Whenever I feel annoyed or depressed, I run to a class. Some of the things that people are now trying to get into in other areas of life, through psychoanalysis and est . . . dancers have been into all along. They can always find their physical and emotional centers. . . ."

According to Gilda Marks, who has the largest dance and exercise school in California, "Everybody's interested in movement these days, regardless of what it is." And that means everybody. Fred Kelly, who started out with his brother Gene, as a "modern dancer," has one tap class in his Oradell, New Jersey, studio in which all the students are grandmothers. His classes are overbooked, as are the courses he teaches at Pace University. Jerry Ames, author of *The Book of Tap* (David McKay), reports that tap class enrollments all over the country have doubled and tripled. The current student enrollment at the Alvin Ailey Dance School in New York is "just over 5,000." Last year it was "closer to 3,000." Elementary classes for adult beginners have been growing steadily over the last two years at the Ellis-Du-Boulay School of Ballet in Chicago. Seven years ago, only three or four tap students a week showed up at the Carnegie Hall International School of Dance (where they also teach ballet, jazz, modern, Hindu, Spanish, Oriental, and Middle-Eastern dance). Now its tap classes seem as crowded as Busby Berkeley production numbers.

The dance boom is reflected in sales of dance gear. "Our business has expanded by 200 percent in the last four years, recession and all," says Walter Seeman, Vice-President of Marketing at Capezio. "The biggest growth has been in leotards and tights—and tap shoes. In January we were back-ordered; we couldn't fill orders for 12,000 pairs of one style of tap shoe, the 1½-inch heel." Meanwhile, at Danskin, leotard sales have gone up 40 to 50 percent and tights sales have risen 30 to 40 percent in the last two years. And Dorothy Hooper, of Danskin, mentioned the incredible and ever-expanding varieties of the contemporary leotard. It comes in colors such as bittersweet and mauve (with matching tights, of course), in satiny nylon or stretch cotton, with wrap-around fronts and plunging backs, even with spaghetti straps. Dancewear is often perfect for streetwear. And the dance "look" has really influenced fashion, from snap-crotch body-suits to opaque pantyhose in zingy colors.

Even more fundamental, however, is the "look" of the dancers themselves. "I really think dancing is the fountain of youth," says Zita Allen. And you have only to look at Dame Margot Fonteyn, Martha Graham, and other patron saints of dance—they're ageless! Underlying the whole new dance movement is, of course, the fact that physical fitness is on everyone's mind. And it is just plain more fun to slim or shape up with music than without. "Fun" is the key here. What was "good for you" was once automatically assumed to be unpleasant. You might have been bored to death huffing through Royal Canadian Air Force exercises every morning— but they were *de rigueur*. Guilt was the motivating force. Straight· exercise is about as appealing to the less Spartan of us as castor oil. With dance, however, you're so busy having a good time that you tend to forget that it also happens to be good for you.

For the serious professional, of course, there is a lot of the repetition, the routine, the strain that accompanies any hard work. But dancing, as work goes, is pleasant. The more you move, the more eloquently you move—the better you feel, physically *and* mentally (a sound body can *make* a sound mind). Isadora Duncan described it: "An expression of serenity ... controlled by the profound rhythm of inner emotion ... it broods first, it sleeps like the life in the seed, and it unfolds with gentle slowness ... the rhythm of all that dies in order to live again ... the eternal rising of the sun ... the rhythm of the waves: the rhythm that rises, penetrates, holding in itself the impulse and the after-movement, call and response, bound endless in one cadence."

In Isadora's time, America was not exactly kicking up its heels. Anna Pavlova toured the country. So did the Denishawn dancers. But dance was neither a national pastime nor a national preoccupation. The fact that it is now both, that people now know about dance as the supreme physical tonic and want to partake is due to tremendous efforts made by dancers, dance writers, and dance fans. Doris Hering, a distinguished critic and longtime supporter of the regional dance movement, is Executive Director of the National Association for Regional Ballet (NARB), which, quite naturally, has as its goal another Isadora vision: "I see America dancing, beautiful, strong, with one foot poised on the highest point of the Rockies, her two hands stretched out from the Atlantic to the Pacific, her fine head tossed to the sky, her forehead shining with a crown of a million stars."

The NARB now has 115 member companies. And Miss Hering has engineered a program, funded by the Andrew W. Mellon Foundation, to form a repertoire for NARB members by carefully choosing the best of over 500 works by regional choreographers. So regional innovations, the accents of the South, the Northwest, Texas, are making themselves felt and seen in the national dance picture, even as NARB companies bring the best of dance to areas heretofore untouched by the art.

And it's easier for people to relate to dance today. Although pure, classical ballet flourishes (nothing draws crowds like *The Nutcracker*), the lines drawn between dancing disciplines have blurred. Richard Philip, Managing Editor of *Dancemagazine*, speaks of "a conglomeration, an amalgamation of style." Then, too, there's the superstar phenomenon. Dance heroes may not approach, say, the Mary Tyler Moores of the world in numbers of press coverage, but their presence is felt. Dance fans have always flocked to see their favorites; now, the public-at-large goes to see Mikhail Baryshnikov (in whatever) and talks about it for the next three weeks. General magazines are glomming on to what used to be the nearly exclusive turf of *Dancemagazine* (as in Baryshnikov's appearance on *Time's* cover). *Dancemagazine's* subscriptions have tripled in the last 5 years, and it nimbly keeps up not just with the stars but with the total dance scene.

It publishes reports from everywhere—Akron, Salt Lake City, St. Paul—and on everything from toe-shoe technology to the state of arts funding. ("Dance has become responsible business," reports Richard Philip.) *Dancemagazine* has a regular TV column. In one recent issue, disco was covered right along with Baryshnikov's latest moves. And let us not overlook the influence of television in the dance boom—not that dance is new to television. But serious efforts to translate major dance works into the TV idiom were thwarted by limited interest on the part of producers and the public, and the limited ability of the cameras to capture the performance. Now, all that is changing. *Dance in America* is not only the first prime-time TV dance series, but the first significant effort of television people and choreographers to cooperate in acclimating dance to TV and vice versa. Martha Graham, for instance, rechoreographed parts of her works because they didn't work on camera.

The power of the televised image and of live performances even in the tiniest communities has sent people running to dance classes because they want to be better audiences, to understand what they're seeing. And the fact that disco dancing is probably second only to TV-watching as a national habit has also boosted dance class enrollments, and not only in straight disco classes. Nobody wants to look awkward on the dance floor.

So as a great big disco hit goes, it's time to "get up and boogie"—if you haven't already. Find the sort of dance that suits you and, as they also say a lot in disco: *"Do it!"* Listen to Fred Kelly: "I don't believe in dividing dancing up. There's room for all of it. And the more people dancing, the happier this country will be."

Don't be afraid to shop around before committing yourself to one particular dance routine, teacher, or regimen. Here's a basic repertoire.

Ballet. "Ballet," says Richard Ellis, of the Ellis-DuBoulay School in Chicago, "is absolutely the basis for *everything* in dance. When *West Side Story* came out, teenagers thought it was all gorgeous, free, but those were all highly trained ballet dancers. If you have ballet training, the rest is much easier." That ballet is the backbone of dance and the most highly involved dance form is indisputable. Classical ballet is highly formalized, and it takes extreme discipline to master body movements and positions that don't come naturally. The language of ballet is French (although the art started in Renaissance Italy). You do *arabesques, grand pliés, frappés, passés, glissades* ... All very valuable for future Cynthia Gregorys, you might say—but what's in it for me?

Just this. The discipline itself is not only vital in other

forms of dance but will infiltrate your whole life, if you let it. Secondly, as Edith D'Addario, of the Robert Joffrey School, points out, "It's marvelous for the body, pulls up every muscle." And then, too, once you've tried to perfect even a good fifth position, you will really begin to comprehend what goes into great dancing, the rigors of making it all look so easy, so fluid.

A ballet wardrobe consists of leotards, tights, soft ballet slippers, and, if you're going all the way, toe shoes. Most schools have "pre-ballet," or adult beginner, classes which start with basic steps and lead you gracefully into the ballet routines and terminology.

Modern dance and jazz dancing. The reason these two very separate and distinct forms of dance have been lumped together is that they are both nearly indefinable in general terms. What modern dance is, what jazz is, depends entirely on who's at the head of the class. In the case of modern, the Martha Graham School was asked for some way of summing it up. A quick survey was taken around the studio. Everyone was "nonplussed." Finally, a statement was made: "Modern dance is as stimulating intellectually as it is physically, which is the reason it has caught on at colleges around the country." True. But it's a long way from your average campus "interpretive dance" class ("Okay, now we're going to be trees, growing trees . . .") to the individual techniques developed (highly) by Martha Graham, José Limon, Merce Cunningham, Katherine Dunham, Doris Humphrey, and Charles Weidman.

While everyone in modern dance is free to develop his or her own vocabulary, there are ground rules. Each technique has its own rules. Students of the above-mentioned pioneers perpetuate what can only be described as the most variegated, changing, and psyche-involving type of dance.

You'll need leotards, tights, and, sometimes, soft ballet shoes. Modern dance is often done barefoot, in which case you need footless tights, or tights with "stirrups." A ballet background is useful, but not essential, since modern dance is as disciplined, as rooted in basics, as ballet (in fact, it borrows a lot from ballet).

Jazz dancing, equally difficult to pin down, is a hodgepodge of everything—ballet, modern, American folk, tap, West Indian, flashy Broadway, whatever is going on in the discos, and much more. Again, it depends on your instructor's orientation. You could learn "routines" (à la *Chorus Line*) or be encouraged to interpret the music your way. No previous dance experience is needed for beginning classes, which often warm you up with stretching, and other exercises, and then proceed to fundamental footwork. Jazz shoes are necessary (they're like tap shoes without the taps), although some jazz teachers prefer sneakers. The usual leotards and tights can be replaced by comfortable pants with a lot of "give," and T-shirts.

Tap. "Tap dancing is happy dancing," says Fred Kelly. "It's pretty hard to cry when you're tap dancing." That, and the show-biz connection (recently reinculcated in the American public via *That's Entertainment* and a lot of nostalgia on Broadway) accounts for the current tap craze. "What you get out of it," explains author and teacher Jerry Ames, "depends on your goal. It's exercise without drudgery. There's a joy in being able to make noise legitimately, especially in a city with horns and sirens. It's a tremendous outlet: there's a relaxation that comes after really letting off steam."

There's instant gratification with tap, too. You may not *really* look like Fred Astaire the first time out, but somehow the mere sound of your own feet tapping makes you feel like a star. Then there's the camaraderie of tap classes. The music blares "Give my regards to Broadway" and you're lined up in a group moving in unison around the room. Jerry Ames, comparing the mood in his classes to the reserved atmosphere of even a beginning ballet class, says, "We really get a kick out of each other—so to speak."

For tap, you'll need stretch, or otherwise comfortable pants, a T-shirt (you'll perspire a lot), and tap shoes. You'll also need energy. Although beginners start slowly, heel-toe-heel-toe, then a little arm business, after that, as Jerry Ames puts it, "You're your own drummer."

Belly dancing. This is the only form of dance that's pretty much for women only. No dance background is required, and the requisite dress is usually a leotard, tights, and ballet slippers or low-heeled flexible shoes. What has put belly dancing on the map, coast to coast, is the fact that it tightens the muscles in the abdomen and around the waist because of the constant stretching and contracting of the midsection. But, as taught by Serena in New York City and many professionals elsewhere, belly dancing utilizes every other part of the body as well.

"I'm not a totally ethnic teacher," says Serena. "The dance I've designed glorifies women, and, frankly, Middle Eastern culture does not. Also, in the Middle East, movements tend to be highly repetitive and boring. Authentic belly dancing is not necessarily a full approach to body movements." So, in seeking out a belly-dancing class, don't be sold only on the fact the instructor is a genuine Turk or Iranian (the techniques differ, incidentally, according to country of origin). Sit in and watch before signing up.

Disco. If you want to do the Hustle, the Bust Stop, the Rope, the Fonz, and the Walk, disco schools are bursting out all over. The best formal lessons start with warm-up exercises, as in nonsocial dance classes. But you can also learn by simply going to the nearest disco club and getting in on the action(s). A round-up of disco havens in *New York* magazine mentioned that local teachers go to one particularly hot night spot to pick up the latest moves from the kids on the dance floor. You can do the same. If you feel inhibited remember that everyone else is too busy to worry about how inexperienced you look.

WHAT DANCING DOES FOR YOUR HEALTH

"Dancing is one of the best forms of heart exercise there is," says Leonore R. Zohman, M.D., Director of Cardiopulmonary Rehabilitation at Montefiore Hospital in New York. She urged dancing on a group of male heart patients, who were reluctant at first, thinking it was "women's stuff"; but after she hired an attractive young choreographer to train them, they began to take to it, and after 6 months, not only had their physical fitness improved considerably, but they didn't want to stop! Dr. Zohman gives four reasons why dancing is such a good conditioner for the heart:

1. If the dancing is sustained, vigorous, and rhythmic (what is called "isotonic"), it can raise your heart rate to the proper target zone for conditioning.

2. You can dance at different intensities, to the same music, depending on your physical condition, so over-stressing yourself need not be a problem in order to keep up with others.

3. Dancing allows you to put the joints of your body through their range of motion, using both legs and arms together. This is highly advantageous because (a) you are strengthening body muscles and maintaining your flexibility, and (b) you are using your arms and legs together—infinitely preferable to exercising them separately.

4. Dancing is FUN. It's social, it's co-ed, and the music keeps you going. This means people are much more willing to dance than to do ordinary exercises.

Chapter 38

HOW TO PERFORM BETTER AT ALMOST EVERYTHING

Most of us feel we could do better. We could do more things, learn more, help people more, enjoy life more, if only ... But if only what? Some people put it down to lack of energy, others to lack of time, still others to lack of goal-orientation. Now Dr. Laurence E. Morehouse, founding director of the Human Performance Laboratory at UCLA, and coauthor (with Leonard Gross) of the best-selling *Total Fitness: In Thirty Minutes a Week,* has come up with a blueprint for improved performance that applies to everyone. In his book, *Maximum Performance* (also written with Leonard Gross), published by Simon & Schuster, Dr. Morehouse declares, "There is in every one of us a better performer than we are." And by following certain principles, he believes we can all get there.

How Dr. Morehouse got there is a lesson in itself. "I tried to be an athlete in high school and college," he explained in an exclusive interview, "but although I won various things, I realized I would never be a champion. So I got interested in the science of champions—the science of performing; and what I've done is analyze the principles that make for champions and apply them to everything we do."

According to Dr. Morehouse, our lives are dominated by certain misconceptions about performance which inhibit maximum achievement. He suggests we watch out for the most common ones:

Beware trying too hard. "People feel they must exhaust themselves to do their best," says Dr. Morehouse. "We use words like 'strive,' whereas champions don't behave like this. They don't exhaust themselves. The expression, 'give 150 percent to the effort,' is false because it induces tension so that you're actually working with your brakes on. In order to move fast, you must *relax* more, not work harder."

Beware thinking too much about what you're doing. "We give over-attention to a lot of things in our daily lives. We are too conscious of the protein, carbohydrate, and fat count in our food; all these things already exist in the right proportions in a properly balanced diet. We try to program bowel movements, when they are much better left to natural processes." Dr. Morehouse tells the story of how he taught swimmers to swim to the center of the pool, turn round, and swim back. He practiced the right body movements with his students on dry land first, but when they tried it out in the water, the failure rate was astonishing. Finally, Dr. Morehouse tried a new plan. He simply told the next groups of students to swim to the center of the pool and then swim back. And they did. In other words, your body often knows more than you think it knows. If you think too hard, your body tenses up and performs less well.

Beware feeling calm before a challenge. "Many people feel that anxiety is a negative feeling. That's a misconception. If you feel terrible, you're probably going to perform well. Champions recognize this, and so do stage actors. There's a physiological basis for this fact, and that is adrenalin, the hormone that produces an immediate increase in metabolism and strengthening of muscular contractions. Without it, your performance may go flat; with it, you have the opportunity to excel."

Beware doing the difficult thing first. "If you have a lot to do and try to get most of it done while you're fresh, figuring you can ease off when you're tired, it does not work. Using this burst of energy is insufficient. It exhausts you, so you are too tired to finish the task. The right way to approach a large task is to divide it up into sections, so that each part of the activity is assigned a certain amount of time. That way you pace yourself, and come to the end without fatigue.

"If, however, you are learning something new, you should do the simple things first. This is very important. For instance, suppose you're going to learn the serve in tennis, which for a lot of people is very, very difficult. It's made up of various components, and one of them is tossing the ball up to the proper height and position. If you are shown how to toss the ball and find you can do it quite easily, then drop that and go on to the next move. If you simply keep on practicing the toss, you will become fatigued, start doing it awkwardly, and then develop bad habits."

Beware comparing yourself with others. "American culture is highly competitive and we're conditioned from earliest days in school to get the grades, to win the races, to look better than the next person, and so forth. This competitive culture is what has made America great, in some respects. But it is also inhibiting for many people. They look at others who appear to be more successful than themselves, and become discouraged and depressed. Comparisons are meaningless. Almost everyone can find someone more awkward than he or she is, and someone more talented. Each person should view his own performance in terms of his wants, needs, limitations, and gifts.

"If you feel you are not functioning well, then you must ask questions. People waste time doing things that they say are satisfying, making beds for example. I could take 15 minutes to make a perfect bed. I could get a kick out of getting all the corners right, no wrinkles anywhere. But I could get all four beds in our house made in 7½ minutes. They would still be pretty good beds, and I would then have time to do other things. We tend to rationalize our time. But comparing the way you spend your time with other people will not help you. The only comparison that is rewarding is this one: *When you do something better today than you were doing it yesterday.* That is the greatest reward of all."

THREE WAYS TO PERFORM BETTER

From his studies with champion athletes, Dr. Morehouse has come up with useful tips to train body and mind to do their best:

1. Keep moving. "Movement keeps you sharp. If you stay at one repetitious task for a long time, it gets boring, you begin to slow down, and it takes you twice as long. Brain circulation depends on pressure of the blood flow. Your working environment should be structured not for comfort but for activity. Your daily program should involve different things."

2. Take a real midday break. "Continuity of work hurts performance. You need time in the middle of the day for personal recuperation from the morning as well as preparation for the afternoon. Try to remove yourself from the place you spent the morning and from the people you were with as well. You need a real break to make transitions from old to new activities."

3. Practice dynamic relaxation. "The idea behind dynamic relaxation is to become aware of your present tension level, deliberately increase that level, then diminish it until you feel loose and wobbly, finally bringing the tension level back to a degree that allows you to perform at your best. Here's a way to do it while walking:
"While you are walking, first of all make yourself tense. Tighten up your arms, legs, neck, so that you are walking very stiffly. Then, as you take these stiff steps gradually let this tension drain away until you're so relaxed that you start to wobble. At this point, bring your tension back up to the walking level at which you can function best. If you were

tense, this will be several notches lower than the level at which you began."

This exercise can be done during any movement, such as running, swinging a golf club, jogging, cleaning house. When you finish your exercise, your body is freewheeling and you are in control of your tension.

Chapter 39

SLEEP—THE WAY TO A HEALTHY LIFE

Most people now know that there are two types of sleep, REM (Rapid Eye Movement, or Dream) and non-REM, that these two states of sleep alternate throughout the night about every 90 minutes, and that we need both types of sleep for physical and mental well-being. But did you know that there are two types of tiredness that are directly related to these two states of sleep?

WHAT TIREDNESS MEANS

"Tiredness is not easy to study," explains Dr. Ernest Hartmann, Director of the Sleep and Dream Laboratory, Boston State Hospital, and Professor of Psychiatry, Tufts University School of Medicine. "But I feel that there are two distinct kinds of tiredness. One comes after physical activity, when you have not been very emotionally or intellectually involved, but it's been a day of sport or physical action. This kind of tiredness feels quite pleasant, and means that you usually fall asleep quite quickly. In children, this simple tiredness is just a "wearing out" without mental involvement, and also means that they fall asleep quickly.

"The second kind of tiredness is probably much more common in our civilized world. This is a mental and emotional tiredness that usually comes after a day of stress or worry. This is characterized by a generally unpleasant feeling—you become irritable, angry, overwhelmed by things around you, depressed, and so on. There are physical manifestations, also—your muscles become tense, you have headaches. And unfortunately, this is a tiredness from which you do not necessarily fall asleep easily. You will lie in bed worrying—tense—too tired to go to sleep. This is particularly noticeable in children; this kind of tiredness makes them scream and become infantile and it's more difficult to get them to go to sleep. This kind of tiredness also seems to make adults regress—you become childishly cross, oversensitive, like a spoiled child."

It is Dr. Hartmann's conclusion, after much study, that for the first kind of tiredness, the physical tiredness, you mainly need non-REM, or slow-wave sleep; and for the second, you need REM, or dream sleep.

This immediately leads to the next conclusion—that sleep has two different but connected restorative functions.

HOW SLEEP RESTORES YOU

"The first restorative function is *body* sleep," explains Dr. Hartmann. "The body having worn out its musculature, or the tissues having been burned up, slow-wave sleep may play a role in restoring these muscles and tissues as well as preparing you for dream sleep. The other kind of sleep— dream sleep—seems more to have a restorative function for the *brain*, for knitting up the 'ravell'd sleave of care,' in Shakespeare's most apt expression—integrating material that has been left over from the day, for instance. It's not pure memory reorganization. It's more like this—if something happened during the day that has emotionally stirred you and brought up old memories and pulled things out of place, unfiled and a little disturbing, sleep not only restores, it also integrates the day's happenings.

"We have noticed, for instance, that if you are particularly worried or under emotional stress, you tend to need more sleep—or at least sleep more—to integrate these difficulties. When things are going well, you sleep less. You then have less need of the restorative qualities of sleep."

HOW TO USE SLEEP

"Since sleep has these integrating, restoring qualities, why not take advantage of it?" asks Dr. Hartmann. "If you have to write a paper, for instance, or get some complicated work done, don't try to do it before you go to sleep, but arrange it, look over the material, and have it in your head before sleep, and you'll find in the morning that the work comes much more easily.

"We have observed that creative people particularly tend to use sleep for these helpful, clearing-the-head qualities. Therefore certain creative people tend to need *more* sleep because they use it more. Practical people are often short sleepers because they work so efficiently and organize their time so well during the day that they do not need to 'waste time' organizing themselves while they sleep."

HOW LONG YOU SHOULD SLEEP

The average person still tends to think of sleep in terms of how many hours he should sleep. But a man can sleep 3 hours a night and wake up feeling perfectly refreshed. And too much sleep can be bad—it deconditions the body *too* much. So you see, it's not the *amount* of sleep you should be thinking about, but the *quality* of it—the balance of REM and non-REM sleep banishing your two types of tiredness and integrating and restoring your mental processes.

Perhaps knowing that sleep has these restorative functions will help you if you find it difficult to fall asleep. For as Dr.

Hartmann says, "If you really believe in sleep, and believe that it will help you in this way, then you won't worry but will fall asleep quite easily."

AND NOW ... *HOW TO GET TO SLEEP*

You know the feeling—climbing into bed after a long day, looking forward to putting your head on the pillow and drifting off into a wonderful, deep, long, soothing sleep, and instead lying there with your head in a whirl, your body tense, waiting in vain for the gift of sleep to come.

Well, you cannot buy sleep. You cannot coax it, cajole it, even trick it into casting its spell over you. But you *can* practice certain routines that may bring sleep a little closer to you—routines that doctors in sleep laboratories in Boston, Philadelphia, and New York have discovered can really help you fall asleep. Some of their suggestions are completely new ideas—others are old wives' tales with a new twist. But one of them might work on you that sleep-inducing magic everyone longs for.

Relaxation

"The basic reason many people can't sleep is some type of muscle tension," says David Davis, director of a private sleep laboratory in New York City and consultant to Mount Sinai Hospital. "The first sign of anxiety, hostility, or fight-or-flight, right from primitive times, is expressed in your facial, neck, and jaw muscles. Next time you become tense or hostile, notice how it first manifests itself—you clench your teeth and tighten your jaw muscles. You'd be surprised how many people try to go to sleep at night like this.

"When you go to bed, to relax, let your jaw hang down." Unclench your jaw, consciously, and fall asleep. (Notice how people who fall asleep sitting up often end up with their mouths hanging open—utterly relaxed.) The key to breaking the muscle tension that stops you from sleeping is relaxing the muscles.

Sleep-food

You have probably heard that a hearty meal makes you drowsy because the blood leaves your head and goes to the stomach to help digestion. Well, that's completely false, according to Dr. Ernest Hartmann. He, and many of his colleagues, believe this drowsiness is actually caused by an amino acid, L-tryptophan, in foods such as meat, cheese, milk, and eggs. It's in everybody's diet to some degree, and most people take 1–2 grams of it every day. When L-tryptophan is taken into the body, it is converted into serotonin, a brain chemical that affects sleep. (It appears to be the ratio of L-tryptophan to other amino acids that creates this effect.) "A high-protein meal of meat, cheese, or eggs—and a glass of milk—contains enough L-tryptophan in pure form to get you to fall asleep," says Dr. Hartmann. "The best source of L-tryptophan is turkey meat—that may be why people tend to fall asleep after Thanksgiving dinner! In our studies we found that a dose of 1 gram of L-tryptophan will cut down the time it takes to fall asleep from 20 to 10 minutes in our laboratory conditions. Of course, we isolated it and gave it in its pure form—in food it competes with other amino acids—but one hopes that one day it can be offered as a sleep inducer at your drug store. Its great advantage is that not only do you get to sleep sooner, but you do so without the distortions in sleep patterns that are produced by most sleeping pills. For now, a high-protein meal or snack before you go to bed may help induce sleep."

Bedtime drinks

Warm Milk. From what has been said about L-tryptophan, it is clear that milk, which contains L-tryptophan, is a sleep inducer. Warm milk also has a soothing effect.

Chamomile Tea. This has a long tradition of being a relaxing and soothing sedative drink. But more scientific proof has recently emerged. Lawrence Gould, MD, and colleagues, writing in the *Journal of Clinical Pharmacology*, described a series of tests run to measure the effect, if any, of chamomile tea on cardiac patients. They found that the tea had no significant *cardiac* effects but that "a striking hypnotic sleep-inducing action of the tea was noted in ten of twelve patients. This was particularly striking since the patients normally found it very difficult to fall asleep." So chamomile tea must be reckoned with as more than just a folk tale.

Alcohol. This is a central nervous system sedative—"it puts the higher brain center to sleep," explains Dr. Joseph Mendels, former Director of the Sleep Laboratory, Veterans Administration Hospital, Philadelphia, and Professor of Psychiatry, University of Pennsylvania. "It is a very good sedative and many people will take a small tot of something before they go to bed; and while one doesn't want to recommend this as a routine for everybody, it may be less pernicious than some of the sleeping medications people take."

Sounds

"Rhythms, such as the sounds on a train, have a hypnotic effect and are aids to sleep," says Dr. Mendels. "It is the monotony of it—anything monotonous is sleep-inducing. For instance, some people had trouble getting their three-year-old child to sleep. They noticed that if there was some rhythmic noise in the background, the child tended to drift off. They found the best way of inducing this noise in the house was by having a vacuum cleaner running. This made the child go to sleep, but it wasn't doing their vacuum cleaner any good. So in the end they made a tape recording of the vacuum cleaner and that became the soporific for the child!

"If you can find a monotonous noise or rhythm to play at night, this may well help you."

Another recent sound discovery was made by an obstetrician at Tokyo's Nippon Medical College. To calm babies in order to examine them, he placed a tiny microphone inside the uterus of several pregnant women and recorded their internal body sounds. When he played back the amplified sounds to groups of screaming infants, almost every single one stopped crying and then dropped off to sleep! The sounds have now been produced in Japan by Toshiba-EMI on a record and cassette, entitled "Lullaby Inside Mum"—a great success with new parents to get babies to go to sleep! (Capitol Records has released it in this country.)

Exercise

"For most people who are in good health, if you go out and exercise to the point once a day or once every other day where you can raise your heart beat and work up a good sweat, you'll find that within a few days you'll need less sleep and you'll sleep better," declares Mr. Davis. "This is not to say that every night just before you go to bed you should run around the park. The exercise should be in the morning or early evening, or whenever it's convenient during the day."

Beds and pillows

Beds are a question of personal taste—there is no rule about them. "What you must do is find what is most comfortable for you," says Dr. Mendels. "The most important thing in bed is not to toss and turn. If you are restless, sit up, turn the light on, and read for a while, or get up and do something else. Tossing and turning tends to aggravate the cycle of not sleeping—you become more tense and make the situation worse."

Mr. Davis suggests that if you are not sleeping, take away your pillow. "Taking away your pillow may help you relax your neck muscles." Relaxing your neck is the crucial part, however you do it. The Japanese for instance, sleep on woodblock pillows, which may be their way of relaxing their necks.

Napping

There are people who can nap for just a few minutes and

wake up feeling rejuvenated. Other people nap and wake up feeling terrible. "The best explanation for this is that we have an inherent rhythm in our makeup. We have a cycle of REM or non-REM sleep, each occurring every 90 minutes or so. Now it seems this cycle not only occurs at night but also during the day—for the full 24 hours in fact. Look at the average office routine: A person comes to work at 8:30 or 9:00; an hour and a half later he stops for a coffee break. Then he goes back to work and another hour and a half it's lunchtime. He comes back and at 3:00 o'clock there's another break. Without knowing what we are doing, we have organized our lives to a rhythm. (Jet lag is a perfect example of what happens when that rhythm is disturbed.)

"If you have a nap at the right point in your cycle, then it is very refreshing. If you wake up at the wrong phase in the rhythm, you feel terrible. If you *do* wake up at the wrong time, all you have to do is go back to sleep to finish the cycle."

Sleeping pills

The last resort. Every doctor consulted agreed on the imperfections of sleeping pills. What many regularly pre-scribed sleeping pills do is disrupt your cycle of sleep, so that your REM sleep is often considerably reduced. The effect of this is that when you *stop* taking the pills, you get what doctors call a "rebound"—that is to say, you spend 40 or 50 percent of the night in REM sleep. "It is as though you were making up for all that REM sleep you were deprived of when taking the pills," says Dr. Mendels. "This means you may start having REM (dream) sleep within a few minutes of falling asleep—and the dreams that you have then have a more nightmarish quality than usual. So you wake up in the morning feeling that you've had a terrible night, and have to go on the pills again!"

It's a vicious circle. So if you can possibly use one of the other aids suggested here, it would be much better for you.

(Unfortunately, the people who use sleeping pills the most tend to be older. They are people who do not realize that the older you get, the less sleep you need.)

There is a system about falling asleep which, if you can achieve it, is going to help you fall asleep more easily and sleep better. If you're reasonably healthy, you have done a little exercise, your mind is at rest, and your body is relaxed—then the great boon of sleep *will* come to you. It's all in the mind. Even going-to-bed routines can help—the way you take off your makeup, brush your hair, settle into bed—these little rituals can calm you down. So if you start being aware of all your preparations for sleep—and maybe use one of the aids suggested here—then you'll soon be at ease with "tired nature's sweet-restorer, balmy sleep!"

Chapter 40

YOUR OWN HOME SPA—THE BATH

Plunging into the bath is one of today's treasured activities—one of the few pleasures left that are free! One reason why we do it, as Desmond Morris points out in *The Naked Ape,* is for grooming purposes. We like to keep our fur clean. "This is rare, in other primates," he adds, "although certain species bathe occasionally, but for us it now plays the major role in body cleansing in most communities."

But people today are understanding more and more the therapeutic effects of bathing. "Millions of water treatments are administered yearly," says Dr. Anna Kara, Director of the Physical Medicine and Rehabilitation Department, Saint Clare's Hospital, Denville, New Jersey, and Assistant Clinical Professor in Medicine (Physical), Cornell University Medical College, addressing the Sixth International Water Quality Symposium. "It must be doing something right."

There are three ways in which water works as a healer, according to Dr. Kara.

1. Heat. "Water is an excellent medium to apply heat to the body. Raising the temperature has the physiologic effect of increasing the metabolic rate. This increases blood flow, which in turn increases the supply of oxygen, various nutrients, antibodies, hormones, and so forth. Heat also has analgesic and sedative effects."

2. Buoyancy. "Archimedes found that a body immersed in fluid is acted upon by a buoyant or lift force equal to the weight of the displaced fluid. This static lift force acts through the center of buoyancy, which is the center of gravity of the displaced volume. In other words, a person immersed up to the neck in water experiences an apparent loss of nine-tenths of his weight. Thus, if you have painful weight-bearing joints, you will usually find it very comfortable to stand and move in water. Those with poor leg muscles will be able to support such a small weight. If you have weak muscles, exercising in water becomes much easier than exercising in air." (For water exercises, see page 367-369.)

3. Massage. "A whirlpool bath (or shower with nozzle heads that project water strongly enough) can act as a massage on tired or painful muscles and joints."

Dr. Kara believes that exercises in water are of great value for the increase and maintenance of mobility of joints as well as strengthening the muscles. "If you practice moving and flexing every joint in your body *in* the water, it will maintain the range of motions in your joints so you won't stiffen up. This is particularly recommended for arthritic patients." The feeling of weightlessness is also relaxing.

"The temperature of the water will help diminish pain," says Dr. Kara. "But do not make the water too hot—just above body temperature is preferable if you are totally immersing your body. If, however, you are concentrating on only one part of the body, say your neck or shoulders, then hotter water would be more beneficial."

There are, of course, chemical additives to water that are also held to have therapeutic value. Many spas use this form of treatment. "The restful atmosphere and relaxation of warm baths seem to favor release of tension and to counteract the stresses of daily living," she concludes. So into the bath, everyone!

WATER, YOUR SKIN AND COSMIC FORCES

Almost 65 percent of your body weight is water. This water acts as a lubricant for limbs, joints, and blood supply—just as the lubricant in a car engine keeps it running smoothly. In short, according to Dr. Laurence E. Morehouse, "water is the most important thing you take into your body. Fat doesn't contain much water. Water comes out of muscle and blood. This is why diets that take off water are so harmful, and why, if you go on a total fast, it is not lack of food you die of, but dehydration."

Keeping this vital water in your body is the function of the skin. Without the water barrier provided by skin, you would dry up. However, social customs being what they are, you are going to be much more interested in how to keep your skin moist (and therefore beautiful) than your body. So here is Dr. Diane G. Tanenbaum, Associate Professor of Dermatology, New York University, and Attending Physician, Lenox Hill Hospital, to explain some rather surprising facts about water on skin.

"Water is what keeps the skin young-looking and smooth," she says, "It acts, as in all of our body, as a lubricant. As we get older, we lose moisture both in our bodies and in our skin, which makes the skin dryer. (Aging skin means that the substance of the skin itself deteriorates, however—it has nothing to do with the water loss.)

"To keep your skin supple, therefore, you need to add moisture. But here is the surprising thing: *Water applied externally to the skin tends to dry it.* This is because when externally applied water meets the moisture in the skin, the elements contained in both tend to equalize, creating a balance—a natural process known as osmosis. And when these elements are sucked out of your skin, water comes with them, thus drying the skin. Hard water, being more full of chemicals and minerals, is the worst offender. Distilled water should cause the least drying.

"In order to prevent this problem, when you apply water to your skin, you should apply oil, too, to postpone evaporation and keep the water in. Most moisturizers on the market, which are oil and water emulsions, do exactly this. It is also possible to moisturize the skin effectively by putting water on it and then immediately applying petroleum jelly, which acts like a sealant for the water.

"Oily-skinned people often have better lubricated skin for the same reason—the oil keeps the water in. This does not mean, of course, that an oily-skinned person does not ever have dry skin. In fact, dry skin is sometimes the result of oily skin: dandruff, for instance. Oily skin (or scalp) does not flake in the normal way, but in large clumps. You may notice this in certain parts of your face at certain times."

There are three main enemies of a moist skin: prolonged exposure to sunlight (which is directly correlated to wrinkling), too much exposure to harsh soaps and detergents, and exposure to overheated rooms.

Drinking lots of water, according to Dr. Tanenbaum, does *not* help dry skin. "It goes straight to the kidneys—that is why people with kidney infections are asked to drink a lot of water: It works as a cleanser. Water has also been known among water addicts (those who drink gallons of water a day) to produce a 'high'—in other words, it goes to the brain!"

According to biologist Lyall Watson, our brains are already 80 percent water, which he thinks links us more closely to cosmic forces (the rhythm of the moon, sun, and earth) than we realize. "Every drop of water in the ocean responds to this force," he says in his book *Supernature*, "and every living marine animal and plant is made aware of the rhythm." So why not us? Furthermore, according to Elaine Morgan in *The Descent of Woman*, the human race was in fact once an aquatic species (hence, so some people say, the salt in our sweat).

So you see, the problem of a well-moisturized skin is a mere drop in the ocean beside all the other wonderful mysteries surrounding the human body and the elixir of life—water.

EIGHT WAYS TO TONE UP IN THE BATH

The waters of the bath are restorative. The tub provides a setting for the transition between day and night, office and home, solitude and socializing. Above all, bathing is a way of treating yourself kindly, an opportunity to loll for a few dreamy moments in warm, buoyant physical splendor. Without detracting from the essential enjoyment of this experience, Barbara Pearlman, an exercise expert, has developed a set of eight exercises incorporating gentle, slow-stretching movements, which she says will enhance the benefits of the bath. "While you're in the tub, you might as well do something for your body. These exercises, if done regularly, are helpful to the common problem areas—legs, buttocks, abdomen, upper arms, and neck." You can repeat them as many times as you want, depending on how much you want to stretch. If you have had no activity during the day, you might want to use more of your time in the tub for stretching.

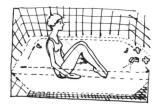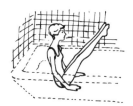

1. Sit with knees bent, toes and fingertips on the floor of the tub. Keeping your stomach muscles contracted, slowly extend both legs outward and upward until they are straight. Hold for two slow counts, then resume original position. Repeat 8 times. (Good for legs, abdomen.)

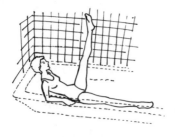

2. Lean back on your elbows. Extend one leg in front and the other upward. Circle the lifted leg in an outward direction. Repeat 12 times on each side. (Good for legs, abdomen.)

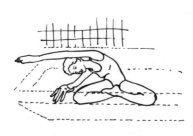

3. Face rim of tub. Sit with ankles crossed, hands resting on rim. Keeping the right hand on tub, arch the left arm overhead (palm facing upward upward) as you simultaneously bounce the torso to the right four times. Return center and repeat to the left. Be sure to keep buttocks stationary while stretching to the side. Repeat 20 times. (Good for arms, waist.)

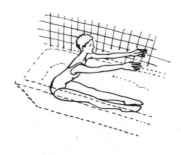

4. Sit with straight back, legs extended in front, arms extended at chest level, palms facing inward. Stretch torso forward in a gentle to-and-fro motion. Repeat 16 times. (Good for back, buttocks, thighs.)

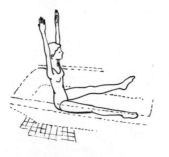

5. Sit with legs extended in front, arms raised overhead. Keeping the back as straight as possible, lift and lower legs alternating sides. Try to raise leg above water level, keeping knees and back straight. Repeat 16 times. (Good for stomach, legs.)

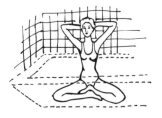

6. Sit facing rim with feet crossed at the ankles, hands clasped behind head. Slowly bring elbows together as head simultaneously drops forward. Hold for three counts, then open elbows to original position. Remember to exhale as you lift. Repeat 15 times. (Good for neck, shoulders, arms, bosom.)

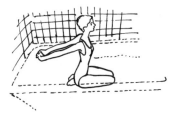

7. Sit on heels with hands clasped behind body. Take two slow counts to raise arms while keeping the torso stationary. Then slowly release. Repeat 10 times. (Good for arms, bosom, shoulders.)

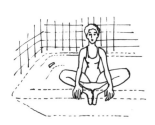 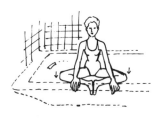

8. Sit facing the tub rim, hands on rim, soles of your feet together. Force the knees downward, hold for five counts, and then release upward. Repeat 12 times. (Good for inner thighs.)

Note: All exercises should be done with a rubber tub mat.

"You don't need an oversize tub to perform them; a standard one will do. The magic ingredient is water. The more there is in the tub, the more rigorous the exercises become because of the resistance. It should be *warm,* not hot, which is drying for the skin and enervating to the body," Mrs. Pearlman warns.

If faithfully followed, she adds, these maneuvers will not only make you feel good (by her definition this means having more stamina, energy, greater command over the body) but help you look good, too.

"Put some herbs in the bath, or some kind of bath softener; have some soft music on and start today."

FIVE TOWEL EXERCISES FROM LARRY LORENCE, DIRECTOR, GALA FITNESS

If you failed to get to your exercises *in* the bath, how about having a little fun and flexibility *out* of the bath—yet without moving further than your towel rail!

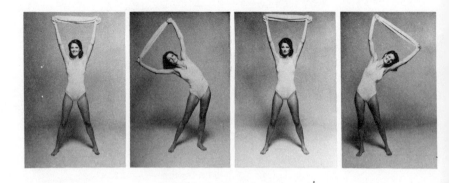

1. *Waistline*
Stand legs apart, hold the towel by outstretched arms above head—bend from side to side.

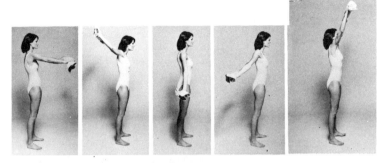

2. *Suppleness of shoulders and stretching*
Hold towel in front in both hands, shoulder width apart (or wider)—raise arms above the head and behind the back—bring the towel over the head and in front again.

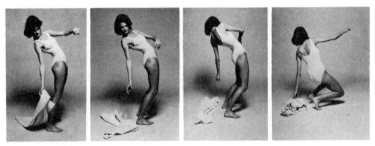

3. *General Suppleness*
Stand with legs apart, hold towel in one hand. Now turn to the right and put down towel behind heels. Next, straighten up, turn to the left, and then pick up towel. Do this exercise three times, then change direction and do it three times the other way.

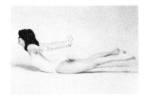
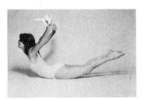

4. *Back*
Lying on stomach on floor, towel behind the back held by both hands with arms outstretched backward, slowly raise legs, arms. Hold 3 seconds—lower.

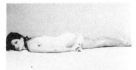

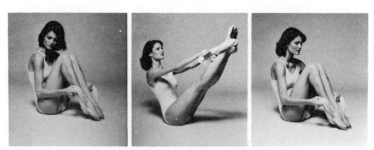

5. *Legs*
Sitting, hold the towel in both hands, put your feet on the towel (with knees bent)—then straighten legs—bend—repeat this exercise 10 times.

Part Five

A HEALTHY MIND

Recognition of the connection between body and mind is becoming more and more a part of modern medicine. A healthy mind seems now to be an essential ingredient in all prescriptions for a healthy life. In this section, doctors and psychological experts suggest various mental techniques you can use to cope with everyday problems, and that will help you and your family get more out of life.

Chapter 41

HOW TO BE HAPPY WITH WHO YOU ARE

If someone asks you, "Are you happy?" what do you say? Many people go through life with the external signs of success—a good job, a nice house, a healthy family—yet experience vague, nagging feelings of dissatisfaction that cannot be articulated. What's wrong? America is supposed to be the richest country in the world. We enjoy many of the qualities of the good life. So why isn't everybody happy?

A man who has devoted most of his life to this problem is psychoanalyst and philosopher Erich Fromm. He is the same age as this century, and through the years he has studied people's worries, fears, hopes, and beliefs, refining and shaping his theories, until now they seem to have come together in one great summary of his vision. He believes that there are two modes of human life. Having and Being. It is living in the "having" mode that makes people unhappy, he feels. Our hope for the future is to change that outlook.

You might think Erich Fromm would be a daunting person, in light of his incredibly distinguished career as doctor and author. Not at all. He is small, frail, and gentle, with bright blue eyes. He talks patiently and generously in a quiet, lightly German-accented voice, the fragility of his manner contrasting with the strength of his ideas.

"Modern man defines himself as 'I am what I have,'" he explains. "Our whole security lies in the fact of having; and since we're insecure, we want to have more and more. This is shown in the development of language. There are many so-called primitive languages which do not have a word for 'I have.' They express it some other way, such as in Semitic languages, by saying 'Something is to me.' The interesting thing is that only later on, with the increase of private property, a new word, 'to have,' was invented.

"I'm a psychoanalyst; so people come to me and say, 'I have insomnia, I have problems, in spite of the fact that I have a nice husband, a nice house, and a car.' Even fifty years ago I can remember a different language: People would say, 'I feel uncomfortable, I am unhappy, I'm unhappily married.' Now we 'have' problems. But that's impossible. One can have a pound of butter, yes. But one cannot have spiritual, mental, or intellectual things. They are inner activities that you experience."

Dr. Fromm then gives an example of how we think in terms of having things. He quotes a haiku by the seventeenth-century Japanese poet, Basho:

> When I look carefully
> I see a little flower blooming
> By the hedge!
> [The exclamation point signifies joy.]

Then he quotes a poem by the nineteenth-century poet, Tennyson:

> Flower in a crannied wall,
> I pluck you out of the crannies,
> I hold you here, root and all, in my hand,
> Little flower ...

"Tennyson has to *have* the flower," Fromm points out, "in order to understand it. The Japanese is content to look at it, to find an inner image of the flower, to relate himself to it without destroying it for the purpose of studying it."

What Dr. Fromm is expressing is of course not unfamiliar. Most of us are aware of our affluent society, the materialist age, our consumerism, and other clichés of the twentieth century. We are aware also that all this material success does not seem to be fulfilling its promise. Happiness evidently is not the second car, the Caribbean cruise, the diamond ring. We may not stop wanting those things, but after the instant gratification, so what? You buy a new dress, love it, wear it, and then want another one. And so it goes.

Oddly enough, Fromm finds some of the attitudes engendered by our affluent society encouraging. "There is a great chance for us," he said. "And I think it's greater in the United States than in any other country in the world. The United States has achieved almost the highest order to give people what they want. Yet today many people have found that this doesn't make them happy. A sailboat hasn't made them happy; a private plane hasn't made them happy—they are the same uneasy, anxious people. If you talk to them, even if they repress the fact, they sense that it's true. Now that is why I say there is a chance.

"You see, people in so-called socialist countries still believe what our grandfathers believed, that if they have a car they will be happy. In Russia or Poland, you would be considered a fool if you suggested they might be better off without private cars. I gave a lecture at the Academy of Science in Warsaw and suggested this, and I have never in my life met with such a stony, hostile silence. Yet it is different for Americans. We have become skeptical. We have started questioning."

Probably the first real questioning began in the sixties, when young people all over America began turning on the old social conventions, freeing themselves from materialist patterns they no longer found helpful, searching for new ways to live happily. They were looking for what Dr. Fromm calls "spiritual content." Today, we are still looking for that content—along a road that Fromm feels may be misleading. You must have noticed the number of gurus popping up everywhere, and the human potential movements that profess to help people find themselves. It's very characteristic of Americans to want to rush out and find a person or credo that will solve everything instantly. Fromm thinks that this leads only to disappointments.

"We tend to be active because we feel we should be active," he says. "If we are not doing things all the time, we feel anxious. Many people cannot sit still for 5 minutes without getting nervous or jittery. So our term of activity means busyness. If somebody said to me, 'What did you do yesterday?' And I said, 'Well I just sat for 3 hours thinking nothing and just feeling myself, the air, who I am,' the other person would probably think I was slightly crazy.

"But the original sense of 'activity,' in the humanist tradition, was 'inner aliveness.' Many great philosophers believed that the highest form of activity is contemplation. Activity means an expression of man's forces, of man's gifts. As a philosopher said, 'People should not consider so much what they are to *do,* as what they *are.*'"

Considering what you are, enjoying 'inner aliveness,' is not easy to come by. You have to make an effort to learn how to be yourself. Dr. Fromm offers this as a start. "Sit still for 15 minutes every day; listen to your breathing; feel it and yourself; and try to think of nothing." This is the first exercise in your attempt to be active in a true sense. "It is difficult to think of nothing," Dr. Fromm says. "Hundreds of thoughts crowd into your mind. But persevere, and you will begin to make progress. We are so busy, we have so much on our minds, that we don't feel anything any more. We are also impatient, so we don't notice what we really feel."

It is during the waiting, the listening and the non-thinking, that you get to know your feelings. "Most people," he says, "at least in my experience, know a lot of what they don't think they know. By which I mean we repress the truth perhaps more than we repress, as Freud thought, our evil strivings. We know a great deal. There is much proof of this. In our dreams we know things that consciously we are unaware of. For instance, you meet a person and are impressed, let us say, by his manners, looks and behavior. You think, 'What a nice person.' Then you have a dream, in which this person tries to kill you. And you say, 'What nonsense.' But after you have dealt with him, you find out that your first impression was wrong, that you were influenced by the wrong things, and it turns out that although that person may not have wanted to go so far as to kill you, he is a scoundrel.

"In general, I think our society requires a good deal of repression of that which we know. It was particularly clear in the case of Richard Nixon. Everybody sensed what the phrase 'Tricky Dick' meant. There was no proof at the time, but people sensed it. We have a sense of things, an unconscious knowledge, that is usually repressed. *The challenge is to follow it, to listen to our own inner responses and become aware of them.*"

Dr. Fromm's own recipe for self-awareness is to practice self-analysis every day, however busy he is, for at least 30 minutes. "I meditate on what I have done, review my own behavior—it's an important thing in my day." It takes time, he warns. There's no easy way. It's not "Find happiness in 12 easy lessons." "To live life successfully you have to *practice* living, every day."

Practicing living takes time, and patience. That is why Dr. Fromm admires people who cook. You cannot hurry a soufflé. "To enjoy cooking is a sign of a life-loving attitude," he told me. "It's a great art that requires patience." Gardeners, too, need patience. A plant takes time to grow. You have to wait and watch. "We know from nature how long a plant grows; we know from nature how long a pregnant woman must wait till the baby is born. There is a lesson to be learnt from nature—that everything takes time, everything goes slowly, in contrast to the overhurried rhythm of our lives."

When asked whether patience was really a key to happiness—that anything that has to be done with patience indicates that it might be a worthwhile thing to do, Dr. Fromm nods. "Yes," he says, "and that makes me think of a Zen Buddhist story, where a young monk came to his Zen Master to learn Buddhism, and after half a year, he told the Master, 'Master, so far you haven't taught me anything.' And the Master answered, 'Haven't you brought me my tea every morning? And haven't I said, 'Thank you?' "

We are advanced enough, according to Dr. Fromm, to sense that money can't buy happiness. The sad face of J. Paul Getty or the pathetic end of Howard Hughes seem proof enough. "Having" isn't the answer. Surely it's reasonable then to take the next step, as Fromm urges: Learn to be, giving birth to all our potentialities, gifts, talent, simply to the wealth of possibilities with which we are all endowed. If he is right, and happiness is found in the patient process of achieving "inner aliveness," then isn't it worth starting right this minute?

WAYS OF BEING

Being yourself is one of the most difficult challenges in today's hectic world. From Erich Fromm's own examples, here are a few exercises to practice that may help you to sort out your own nature from all the extraneous elements that may be smothering it.

1. Sit still for 15 minutes every day. Listen to your breathing, feel it, and think of nothing at all.

2. Review your own behavior at the end of each day so you get to know yourself better.

3. Trust to your inner responses—you probably know more than you think.

4. Concentrate on activities that demand patience—the rewards will be greater.

Chapter 42

GETTING ORGANIZED

Why do you do one thing rather than another? When you wash your hair or vote for president, what are the processes going on in your head that cause you to act? Why are some people more organized than others? There are a few men today who spend much of their time pondering such questions and Gregory Bateson is one of them.

Gregory Bateson, now in his seventies, has astounded the academic community throughout his life with his revolutionary approach to biology, anthropology, psychiatry, communications theory, genetics, cybernetics, and ecology. His famous "double bind" theory of mental pathology is now part of the psychiatric vocabulary. He has worked at the Veterans Administration Hospital in Palo Alto with schizophrenics, at the Oceanic Institute in Hawaii with whales, with his former wife, Margaret Mead, in Bali and New Guinea, with John Lilly and dolphins, and is currently teaching anthropology, cybernetics, and genetics at Kresge College, University of California at Santa Cruz. Probably the best known of his many papers and books is *Steps to an Ecology of Mind* (Ballantine). He now lives with his wife, Lois, and their eight-year-old daughter in California.

Enormously tall, with a face like a benign hawk, he greets visitors in his large farmhouse kitchen, which overlooks the hills just above Santa Cruz. On the English burled oak table, along with cornflakes, pencils, and a child's sock, the *Oxford Book of Quotations* lies open beside the telephone. On a nearby shelf, the *Encyclopaedia Britannica* sits side by side in a neighborly fashion with gardening and cookbooks. A fish tank gurgles behind him. A cat asks to be stroked. Against this background, the distinguished thinker expounds, in bare feet, with frequent pauses, in an accent redolent of England, where he was born. At the end of a particularly complex idea, he will sometimes give a small chortle, eyeing with satisfaction his perplexed audience.

"Why do we want to be organized? Why do we have this need to control our lives?" He looks at the table. "Terror?" he says at last. "We build on our babyhood in order to make what we are when we are grown-up. When we are babies, we are concerned with very simple, basic things like eating, walking, and balancing. I think it's the terror associated with these things, especially the terror of walking, of loss of balance, of loss of control, that makes us determined to organize our lives.

"As we grow up, we are constantly trying to reaffirm that the world is fairly steady. The Balinese had a very organized civilization and then, in the mid-nineteenth century, the Dutch came. There's a word in Balinese for the time before the Dutch, and the phrase is 'when the world was steady.' So it is important you see, that the body be able to walk—and for us to be able to balance."

There is a pause. The fish tank gurgles.

"There are really two ways in which the human mind adapts," he explains. "If you want to shoot a bird, there are essentially two ways of doing it. One is to aim at the bird with a rifle. You look along the sights of the rifle, you see an error, and you correct it and correct it and correct it until you pull the trigger. That is correcting error in the course of the action, using *feedback*.

"The other is essentially using rules laid down for computation. You see a duck rise at one point from the water, and you watch the direction of his flight and how fast he is going, and you raise a shotgun and go bang. And if you are sufficiently practiced in this, you'll get the bird.

"Let's call this second method *calibration*. It's a different sort of adaptation, in which you are not mainly correcting errors in the action. Rather you are set, like a measuring instrument; you could put screwdrivers, as it were, into your head and fix it so your response to the situation is calibrated—and made as accurate as possible through practice. You therefore have to practice like hell."

He looks up and laughs. "Now," he goes on, "you may ask which method people use in their day-to-day behavior. Well, the answer is a combination of both—and it gets to be quite complicated." He is beginning to enjoy himself. "I worked with a family once where the father never got out of work till 6:30. It took him nearly an hour to drive home, so he never got home till 7:30. But supper was at 6:30, so he was late for supper every night. The system was calibrated to supper at 6:30, and every night his wife blamed him. Neither of them, interestingly enough, suggested changing suppertime. He didn't, I suspect, because at some level he liked to annoy. She didn't because she liked to have him in the wrong.

"Their mental responses went something like this: He looks at the clock, sees he is going to be late, and hurries home on a feedback-correcting-error basis. But he's still out of kilter because the calibration is fixed, and what is needed is another feedback to correct the calibration."

Bateson draws a zigzag in the air, showing the pattern of feedback to calibration to feedback. "How do we get calibrated in the first place?" the visitor asks him finally, in the middle of one of his profound silences, during which he seems quite to have forgotten his surroundings.

"There will always be a tendency to take that which you do and make it into the rule for what you are going to do later. It's the phenomenon of habit. The notion of case law (based on precedent), upon which English law is founded, is an example of this. *The habit phenomenon, or formation of calibrations, is an inevitable part of the human mind. It is how we are constructed.*

"Do you know what a cliché is? I think it was originally a French printer's word. When they print a sentence they have to take the separate letters and put them one by one into a sort of grooved stick to spell out the sentence. But for words and sentences which people use often, the printer keeps little sticks of letters ready made up. And these ready-made sentences are called clichés.

"If the printer wants to print something new, say, something in a new language, he will have to break up all that old sorting of the letters. In the same way, in order to think new thoughts or to say new things, we have to break up all our ready-made ideas and shuffle the pieces."

Bateson is building a picture with the mind as an instrument, which, through society and culture, gets "set" in certain fixed patterns, some useful, and some not. In his book *Steps to an Ecology of Mind,* he gives an example: "Think of the house thermostat in your home. The weather changes outdoors; the temperature of the room falls; the thermometer switch in the living room goes through its business and switches on the furnace; and the furnace warms the room and when the room is hot, the thermometer switch turns it off again ... But there is also a little box in the living room on the wall by which you *set* the thermostat. If the house has been too cold for the last week, you must move it up from its present setting to make the system now oscillate around a new level. No amount of weather, heat or cold or whatever, will change that setting. The temperature of the house will get hotter and cooler according to various circumstances, but the setting of the mechanism will not be changed by those changes—until *you* go and *you* move it again."

But how do you change the setting or calibration in your head? It is surely not a matter of moving a needle on a dial— if only it were. He begins to talk about *practice.*

"I was interviewing a Japanese girl once," he says, "about *respect* in the Japanese family: Who respects whom; who sits where; who opens the door for whom. She gave me beautifully detailed answers for half an hour. Then I asked one more question and she said, in a breathless voice, 'But in Japan we do not respect the father.' I said, 'But what have you been telling me for half an hour?' 'Oh, well, you see, we *practice* respect for the father.' I said, 'Why do you do that?' 'In case we need to respect someone.' "

There is a pause, understandably enough, after that one. "Look down *that* hole," he says. Then he comes to the rescue. "Well, the solution is that *in the West we think of practice as something quite different from how they think of it. We think of it as acquiring a skill which we will then use in a particular situation. They think of practice as changing a person.* We, unchanged, will use the skill as though it were a tool. They change the self by practice: You become the sort of person who is *able* to respect when you *need* to respect someone."

He then mentions the book *Zen in the Art of Archery* by Eugen Herrigel. In it, the teacher asks the student to draw the bow "by letting go of yourself, leaving yourself and everything yours behind you so decisively that nothing more is left of you but a purposeless tension you must practice over and over, for years, and in the process, you become a different person." As the teacher says, "You will see with other eyes and measure with other measures."

In other words, practice seems to be a key to change—not in the sense of "practice makes perfect," but more, "practice makes different." The goal being, as always, to achieve balance. And balance, after all, is a matter of calibration: Without it, you are lost.

"A lot of my students today have no core to hold on to in their lives," Bateson said, pacing up and down across the floor. "They have changed all sorts of thing, such as the role of sex, the uses of hypocrisy, and grading systems. Many of these changes are very good, or at least are backstops against things that had become very bad. But then they are left with what in the Middle Ages was called *accidie*—the idea that nothing is particularly worth doing and there's no particular reason for doing it. It's a formidable thing. They don't have a standard against which to measure themselves."

His wife comes into the room, and listens. "And this refers back to the first question," he says with startling recall. "*You go through life with various calibrations relating to feedback. Sometimes, if these calibrations are based on error, they can get you into trouble. But to have none is to have nothing to correct towards, to establish balance.*"

Another example is the environment, about which Bateson is very concerned. Here again, it is a question of balance, in this case disturbed by man's wrong thinking about the way nature works. We cannot blame "technology," or "the system"; it is our error, in our mental calibrations.

It seems we need rules, both as individuals and as a society—but we must be ready at any time to change the rules in order to achieve balance, both within ourselves and for the world we live in.

Chapter 43

THE GREAT ESCAPE–GETTING OUT OF A RUT

The famous Dr. Edward Jenner was busy trying to solve the problem of smallpox. After studying case after case, he still found no possible cure. He had reached an impasse in his thinking. At this point, he changed his tactics. Instead of focusing on people who had smallpox, he switched his attention to people who did not have smallpox. It turned out that dairymaids apparently never got the disease. From the discovery that harmless cowpox gave protection against deadly smallpox came vaccination and the end of smallpox as a scourge in the Western world.

LATERAL THINKING

We often reach an impasse in our thinking. We are looking at a problem and trying to solve it and it seems there is a dead end, an "aporia" (the technical term in logic meaning "no opening"). It is on these occasions that we become tense, we feel pressured, overwhelmed, in a state of stress. We struggle vainly, fighting to solve the problem.

Dr. Jenner, however, did something about this situation. He stopped fighting the problem and simply changed his point of view—from patients to dairymaids. Picture the process going something like this: Suppose the brain is a computer.

This computer has absorbed into its memory bank all your history, your experiences, your training, your information received through life; and it is programmed according to all this data. To change your point of view, you must reprogram your computer, thus freeing yourself to take in new ideas and develop new ways of looking at things. Dr. Jenner, in effect, by reprogramming his computer, erased the old way of looking at his smallpox problem and was free to receive new alternatives.

That's all very well, you may say, but how do we actually *do* that?

Doctor and philosopher Edward de Bono has come up with a technique for changing our point of view, and he calls it lateral thinking.

The normal Western approach to a problem is to *fight* it. The saying, "When the going gets tough, the tough get going," epitomizes this aggressive, combat-ready attitude toward problem solving. No matter what the problem is, or the techniques available for solving it, the framework produced by our Western way of thinking is *fight*. Dr. de Bono calls this *vertical* thinking: the traditional, sequential Aristotelian thinking of logic, moving firmly from one step to the next, like toy blocks being built one on top of the other. The flaw is, of course, that if at any point one of the steps is not reached, or one of the toy blocks is incorrectly placed, then the whole structure collapses. Impasse is reached, and frustration, tension, feelings of *fight* take over.

Lateral thinking, Dr. de Bono says, is a new technique of thinking about things—a technique that avoids this fight altogether, and solves the problem in an entirely unexpected fashion.

In one of Sherlock Holmes's cases, his assistant, Dr. Watson, pointed out that a certain dog was of no importance to the case because it did not appear to have done anything. Sherlock Holmes took the opposite point of view and maintained that the fact the dog had done nothing was of the utmost significance, for it should have been expected to do something, and on this basis he solved the case. [This and the Dr. Jenner example come from Dr. de Bono's book, *New Think* (Basic Books).]

Lateral thinking sounds simple. And it is. Once you have solved the problem laterally, you wonder how you could ever have been hung up on it. The knack is making that vital shift in emphasis, that sidestepping of the problem, instead of grappling with it head-on. It could even be as simple as going to a special part of the house which is quiet and restful or buying a special chair, an "escape" chair, where you can lose your day-to-day preoccupations and allow your computer to reprogram itself and become free to take in new ideas, see things in a different light.

Dr. A. A. Bridger, psychiatrist at Columbia University and in private practice in New York, explains how lateral thinking works for his patients. "Many people come to me, trying to stop smoking, for instance," he says. "Most people fail when they are trying to stop smoking because they wind up telling themselves, 'No, I will not smoke; no, I will not smoke; no, I will not; no, I cannot.' It's a fight—and fighting makes as much sense as telling yourself over and over not to think of what you want. What happens is you end up smoking more.

"So instead of looking at the problem from saying *no,* and fighting it, I show how to reinforce a position of *yes.* I give them a whole new point of view—that you're your body's keeper, and your body is a physical plant through which you experience life. If you stop to think about it, there's something helpless about your body. It can do nothing for itself. It has no choice, like a baby's body. You begin then to find a new way of looking at it—'I am now going to take care of myself and give myself respect and protection by not smoking'—so that not giving yourself respect and protection becomes a deprivation.

"There is a Japanese parable about a jackass tied to a pole

by a rope. The rope rubs against his neck. The more the jackass fights and pulls on the rope, the tighter and tighter it gets around his throat—until he falls down dead as a doornail. On the other hand, as soon as he stops fighting, he finds that the rope gets slack; he can walk around, maybe find some grass to eat ... That's the principle: The more you fight something the more anxious you become—the more you're involved in a bad pattern, the more difficult it is to escape pain.

"Lateral thinking," Dr. Bridger goes on, "is simply approaching a problem with what I would call an Eastern flanking maneuver. You know, when a Zen archer starts to hit the target with a bow and arrow, he doesn't concentrate on the target, he concentrates rather on what he has in his hands, so when he lets the arrow go, his focus is on the end-result of the arrow, rather than on the target. This is what an Eastern flanking maneuver implies—instead of approaching the target directly, you approach it from a sideways point of view, or laterally instead of vertically."

Dr. Bridger has made a shift away from traditional thinking in his practice. "We are finally beginning to realize that many long-term problems can be resolved in short-term ways. People for years have always felt that problems that have been around for a long time will take a very long time to solve. That just does not happen to be so. For instance, when a patient is anxious, fighting a problem, often he can be taught, in one hypnotic session, how to relax and lower his psychic tension. This creates a much more workable feeling-tone for problem solving. While medicines can also lower tension, all medicines, after all, are poisons. Other forms of relaxation, such as transcendental meditation, take a very long period of time to get going. Hypnosis, by contrast, is a safe, quick lateral technique of lowering psychic tension and shifting gears. This increases receptivity for looking at a problem in a new way."

Reminding ourselves we are in a period called an *intermediate impossible* is another useful technique. That is, looking at our current situation in life as only an intermediate step toward something else, so that we don't get bogged down and can go on to the next step. The medical student, for instance, unless he accepted his training as an intermediate impossible, would never get through it. Another familiar example is the harassed mother raising young children—going through the "Terrible Twos." She sees her life as a nightmare—"God, this is going to be the way it is until they are grown up"—as opposed to seeing the "Terrible Twos" as an intermediate impossible. If only she could remind herself that the current situation is intermediate, only a phase, she might relax—if only she could look at her situation laterally, instead of fighting it.

These are difficult questions, and it takes imagination to ask and to answer them. But that is how we change our point of view—being imaginative enough to think up new ideas, find new ways of looking at old problems, invent new methods for dealing with old patterns. Think laterally instead of vertically. Take the *fight* out of our lives. Move Eastward in our attitudes.

"I think the answer lies in that direction," affirms Dr. Bridger. "Take the situation where someone is in a crisis. The Chinese word for crisis is divided into two characters, one meaning 'danger' and the other meaning 'opportunity.' We in the Western world focus only upon the 'danger' aspect of crisis. Crisis in Western civilization has come to mean danger, period. And yet the word can also mean opportunity. Let us now suggest to the person in crisis that he cease concentrating so upon the dangers involved and the difficulties, and concentrate instead upon opportunity, for there is always opportunity in crisis. Looking at a crisis from an opportunity point of view is a lateral thought.

"It's about time we stopped fighting in order to find a solution. Let us float along with the problem so that we can look at it from lateral points of view. Then we can be receptive to new ideas, renew and restimulate our senses, find a new way of living."

How to use lateral thinking

Lateral thinking, in short, is most valuable in those problem situations where vertical thinking has been unable to provide a solution. When you reach that impasse, and feel the fight upon you, quickly reprogram your thinking:

1. Is there any other way the problem can be expressed?

2. What random ideas come to mind when you relax and think about it?

3. Can you turn the problem upside down?

4. Can you invent another problem to take its place?

5. Can you shift the emphasis from one part of the problem to another?

BREAKING ROUTINE

"There are really three kinds of escape," explains Dr. Joel R. Davitz, Professor of Psychology at Teacher's College, Columbia University. "There is the kind of short-term escape, such as when my wife and I run out of steam when writing—we both go down to the basement where I paint and sculpt, and she sews. This occurs when you are functioning at a fairly high level of tension and energy output, then come to a point at which you can't take the tension any more and need to shift activities.

"There's a well-known psychological illustration of this, in which a person is asked to write 'New Jersey Chamber of Commerce' as often as he can until he gives up. He may write it 500 or 1,500 times, but finally he says, 'I can't write any more, not another word, it's quite impossible.' So then, the psychologist says, 'All right. Just sign your name then,' and the person picks up the pen and signs his name. What this exemplifies is a break in activity that reduces tension, changes the previous pattern of behavior, revitalizes, and reactivates.

"This kind of escape takes another form: Rather than switching activities, one switches surroundings—moving from a functional room to a room decorated entirely personally, for instance; from a neutrally colored place to a brightly colored place; from a cluttered corner to a spacious area, or, the extreme example, moving from a city house to a country house. These are all ways, not only of reducing stress and tension, but also of revitalizing and refreshing yourself with new stimulus input. All of us do this, I think, and it is very important.

"Another kind of escape is almost the opposite of that, and is also quite common—escape from boredom. This is not an escape from tension so much as escaping from the emotional reaction of boredom with your life or what you are doing. The use of television is a very common example of how people cope with this kind of boredom—they try to escape by turning to cops and robbers, love stories, sex.

"But there is an altogether different kind of escape, far more important than both of these. This is an escape which is part of psychological growth. It's not escape *from*, but escape *to*.

"In your day-to-day life, there are certain routines and skills that you have acquired and that you must use in order to conduct your activities successfully. In these circumstances, you cannot do too much experimenting or trying out new things. What you have learned in the way of running your house, doing a job, functioning in the community, is a professional skill, and you ought to stick to it if you want to continue doing well.

"But there are certain times in life when you become dissatisfied with yourself as you have been—and these are the periods that are characterized by efforts toward psychological growth. In these periods, you want to escape from the daily routine and responsibilities *in order to try out different parts of yourself*. And it is out of these escapes that we get, during adult life, significant periods of psychological growth.

"The escape can be quite limited. Let us take the stockbroker or banker, for instance, who by virtue of his everyday demands has learned to be a rather controlled and organized person—and this works well with his career. It would not do for him to be very flamboyant. This man may find his escape on the tennis court. Very often, you see a middle-aged professional man turn into a wild man on the court. What he is doing is not just releasing tension, though that is part of it. On the tennis court he can be Jimmy Connors. If he takes a vacation in the Caribbean and instead of his usual three-piece suit takes outlandish costumes, he's not just playing games or being adolescent: He is trying out, in a non-threatening situation, a new aspect of himself.

"A friend of mine recently bought a motorcycle. He has always been a conservative sort of person, and five years ago would have laughed at the idea of leather jackets and helmets. But he drove about on his motorcycle for some time (to the alarm of his family) before giving it up. Now he seems the same, but actually he's quite different. He was shaken up, and has now realigned himself. He has greater acceptance about certain things—for instance, he is much more in touch with his adolescent son. You could regard the process like a kaleidoscope: The pieces are always the same, but if you shake them up they fall into place differently.

"People who make this kind of escape—for instance, taking up painting or sculpture, or going on leave for several weeks or months—usually come back to their ordinary lives. But they come back with a difference. The man who decides to become an artist, for instance, may go back to being a dentist. But having had that experience of working with color, clay, wood, or stone, he goes back to his daily life seeing the world differently. You cannot work at painting without it having an effect on your perspective. Psychologists view it as a spiral—you've gone up the spiral and come to the same position, but higher.

"Without this escape, you would not experience the psychological growth that is so vital to this time of life. Most people do it one way or another, though often it is difficult for family or friends to understand it. Wanting to be a new person can be threatening. Also in our culture there is an underlying feeling of guilt attached to escape—we feel we shouldn't do such things when we are grown-up, though in fact none of us is ever really grown-up. We are always in the process of growing.

"The adolescent goes through a similar kind of growth crisis. He can often afford to take longer-term escapes than the adult; he can have what Erikson calls a 'moratorium,' taking off and traveling, for instance. He needs also to get away from the demanding requirements of daily life to a place where he can try things out for himself.

"So if we take three people at different ages, all making a journey to the South Sea Islands: For the adolescent, it might be a voyage of self-experimentation; for the twenty-five to thirty-five-year-old, it might be a tension reducer, a refresher, and for the forty-five-year-old, it might be an attempt to try out another part of him or herself. All these escapes are useful at different times, but the most important is the one that provides you with a way to discover other parts of yourself, a sure route to psychological growth and greater happiness."

Chapter 44

TALKING IT OVER

We all know it helps to talk things over. Sometimes merely stating a problem aloud inspires a flood of ideas that helps to clarify your thoughts. Having a sympathetic listener is supportive. This act of listening is the basis of modern psychotherapy. In fact, doctors in all branches of medicine believe their most important function in helping a patient get better is lending an ear to personal problems, and maintaining a reassuring manner along with an impartial attitude of interest. This prophylaxis applies equally as well to a simple case of nervous backache as to more complicated anxiety syndromes with no specific symptoms.

When we start life, as children, we're completely open and frank about feelings and say what's on our mind. We never really lose that wish or need to talk out. In our changing society, the traditional figures of wisdom we confide in are fast disappearing. Since one-third of white-collar workers travel geographically as they move up the executive ladder, physical separation between families results in a breakdown of intimate communication. This divides people from people and diminishes the value of parental guidance and experience. Another shrinking corps of listeners are ministers of religion. Apparently people don't turn to clerical ears as they used to. Back in the Depression, there were "listeners" (just ordinary people), who for fifty cents or a dollar did nothing but hear out a person's troubles. More recently, many people have preferred to pay considerably more to shed intimate fears, worries, and problems in the privacy of the analyst's office.

Dr. Bernard Green is one therapist whose office often receives ten people a day. He is a New York psychotherapist who studied at Trinity College, Dublin, and Sussex College, England. He has advised major companies in Europe on matters of industrial psychology and came to America in 1967 to found the International Awareness Center, a research group designed to explore new methods of psychotherapy. He is in private practice and a fellow of the American Society for Psychical Research, and as a lecturer on psychotherapeutic techniques has given papers at professional congresses in Prague, Monte Carlo, and other cities. He is a professional who believes wholeheartedly in the old-fashioned non-professional shoulder of friendship, too, for times when you want to get something off your chest. "We've got to reestablish codes of confidence between friends," he declares. Consider your own circle, people you have known a long time. Surely there exists a person in whom you can confide? Dr. Green's recommendation, in fact, is that you seek out not one but *three* personal confidants. Spreading the load of confidences among three people extends your own involvement with other people's lives and experiences. By doing so, you gain deeper understanding of life, in turn become less critical, more thoughtful, and able to see *yourself* better.

CONFIDENTIALLY SPEAKING

There are three critical areas in life: love and sex; money and work; health and well-being. Never, says Dr. Green, has the need to express feelings on these subjects been greater. "We have more to absorb today, so we tend to block out much more than we ever blocked out before." Because sex, money, and health represent areas in which we experience the most failure and rejection, we're afraid of them and disassociate from them as often as we can, concerning ourselves with other, more trivial matters. Straight talk about love, money, and health brings us in touch with true feelings, which in turn give us direction for real-life situations. For your friendly rap sessions to be more fruitful, says Dr. Green, you must look for your three confidants among friends of the same sex. Confidential exchanges between members of the opposite sex (even marriage partners) are difficult to achieve, he explains, because we have been brought up with the idea that we have "friendship" with the same sex, and another kind of relationship with the opposite sex. "Though some husbands will talk about money and business or their health with their wives, most turn to another man when they discuss sex. There is also a hangover based on the old-fashioned notion that a woman is different and not worthy of confidence—a notion totally wrong and going out."

Selection of three confidants will mark a significant change in your life and that of your confidant. We live at a time when confidential exchanges tend to be feared because respect for privacy is so often violated. Frequently, to say to someone that what you are going to tell him is for his ears alone, is a signal for that person to break your confidence immediately and leak the news. "Talk about people is more interesting than talk about the weather or latest election figures," points out Dr. Green.

THE ART OF BEING A CONFIDANT

To let your friends help you—and for you, likewise, to help your friends—there has to be some understanding of what it takes to be a confidant. There is no need for praise or blame, judgment or any neat advisory to "snap out of it," says Dr. Green. Arguing about what is right, wrong, or silly is equally ineffective. The person talking wants reassurance that his communications are being received. There must not be any interruption, but brief acknowledgments, verbal or nonverbal, are helpful in keeping the conversation going. The listener offers no specific advice, but gently encourages the talker to explore his or her feelings and *shares* the investigation. The confidant's questions, experiences, and illustrative examples aim at illuminating the problem, not at offering conclusions. The object of the exchange is to help the other person come to grips with ineffectual behavior and replace it with a better behavior.

Other psychoanalysts besides Dr. Green have affirmed the positive power of the nonprofessional method. Dr. Lawrence Kubie, an innovative thinker about psychoanalysis, set down in his book *Practical and Theoretical Aspects of Psychoanalysis* the results to be gained, and strongly recommended "talking it out" to ordinary friends before considering formal therapy. He found it offered:

1. Practical support, guidance, and help in life situations.

2. Emotional support, sympathy, encouragement, humor.

3. Reeducation—homely, nonspecific methods of wiser, experienced people helping to reorient a person's attitude.

Modern methods of biofeedback have also proved conclusively that unburdening of problems changes brain waves from delta (worry vibrations) to theta or alpha (relaxed wavelengths). With the brain in a calm position, physical tranquility results, and feelings of well-being and optimism follow. "Many people," says Dr. Green, "try to make tomorrow's dreams or fantasies today's reality—which isn't always possible—and there stems a conflict, and tension." Taking a tranquilizer gives you a temporary lift, then a quick letdown, basically because it doesn't help you to feel your real feelings, Dr. Green points out. Deep conversations can break through character armor and other defenses you put out to the world, and get down to "down" feelings. Such low moods are usually related to anger. To talk about what is making you angry is far more beneficial than suppressing it with a pink tablet.

THE BIG THREE: MONEY, HEALTH, SEX

Love, money, and health are three areas of life related to the "manifest" needs—to feel loved, accepted, acknowledged, secure, and cared for, and to associate with another person in a cooperative effort—all of which are crucial for healthy personality development and functioning. Today, with permissive attitudes and increased eroticism in movies and magazines, sexual performance is more on people's minds than love. "Yet really successful sexual activities are governed by the amount of affection that you have for a person rather than any particular technique," says Dr. Green. "Sex is a combination of warm and loving feelings between two people and it's most satisfying under those conditions." Here's where confidential conversations can help to put fantasies into perspective. For example, when people tend to blow small things out of proportion, a listener can effectively say "so what," "it's nothing," "what difference does it make?" And at the other extreme, confidants can absorb and help clarify deeper sexual conflicts.

When it comes to money and business, you can be overtaken by a need to need, explains Dr. Green. "People may not have such a lack of money or possessions, as a lack of contentment. We inflate the need for money. Does it matter if we don't have the latest car or a villa in the south of France? Money is used as a tool to buy security and love— a new fur or bracelet equals more love." Again, talking and listening can isolate the underlying factors. Examining their credibility often reduces the subconscious drive to get more money and thus the worry of not having enough.

Fear of growing old lurks within everyone. Influenced by young, vibrant heroes and heroines in the news, we are reluctant to face physical maturity, graying hair, and a body of withering strength. No one wants to be "square"; everyone wants to be actively "with it." And there is a psychological bonus to this aim. Mentally, looking and feeling good leads to improved self-esteem. Some people need encouragement in their fitness program and this is where a friend can be helpful. "The role of confidant in the health area is to provide a balance between emotional support and painful truth," says Dr. Green. Any kind of physical self-improvement establishes an emotional "up" and better self-image, "but for the best results it should be done when the subject is in a positive mood and generally feeling good about himself. Good health starts from the inside and moves out." The confidant tries first to change the mental set, then proceeds to encourage action.

RAP-UP

Your confidants shouldn't be expected to tell you what to do, but only to help you arrive at your own decisions. To a great extent, he or she will serve as a sounding board against which you bounce your ideas, hear your inner thoughts. In the process, confusion disperses. Talking out, then, is a miraculous, natural healing process.

Your confidant must be chosen with three points in mind:

—Someone you feel you can trust to keep what you are saying to himself or herself.
—Someone who can listen.
—Someone who has more experience in the subject than you have. The person doesn't necessarily have to be older, but is someone whose views you respect.

Chapter 45

HOW TO CONTROL YOUR WEIGHT, YOUR TEMPER, AND YOUR LIFE

What is responsible for what goes on in your life? Is it you, yourself, or is it external events? Psychological research indicates that people differ quite markedly in the way they attribute the causes of major events in their lives. And it may not surprise you to learn that people who think they themselves are in control of things are usually in much better shape than those who feel they are out of control. In fact, the extent to which people feel they are gaining control over their lives is used as a measure of improvement in psychiatric wards.

Yet not so long ago "control" was considered a bad word. Children were taught to be uninhibited. Parents believed that too much discipline might hinder their offspring's emotional development. Generations of psychiatry have led Americans to be suspicious of restraint or self-control.

But what happened? Could it be that "letting it all hang out" has become old-fashioned? One of the key attractions to the Reverend Sun Myung Moon's followers is his insistence on discipline. The young "Moonies" are rigidly organized by timetables, work assignments, and other forms of social structure that they seem to thrive on. Their lives are under control.

Est, another astonishingly successful movement with the under-thirty-fives, offers a rigorous course in self-discipline. The first day's "training" (note the word) involves sitting for many hours in silence listening to a trainer heap abuse and instruction upon you, during which you may not leave the room, even to go to the bathroom. The est teaching is a basic approach to self-control: "You are responsible for what you are," they tell you. "Irresistible forces are not sweeping you into disasters at home or at work. You are in control of your life and what is, is, because you willed it so." It is precisely this philosophy of returning responsibility to the individual, that has caused est to be so enthusiastically received.

In a recent interview, writer Nora Ephron was asked this question: "Women often want everything. What is everything to you?" She replied, "Everything to me is just very simply being in control of my life."

But how do you get control? How do you impose self-discipline? How can you summon up enough will power to prevent yourself from getting out of control?

The people who probably most often ask these questions are dieters. Losing weight is surely one of the most testing arenas of all for practicing self-control. Peter Herman, Assistant Professor of Psychology at the University of Toronto, has been studying the conditions which affect a dieter's resolve, and what he has discovered may cast some light on that most elusive of human qualities, willpower.

"I believe that willpower is something everybody has," Dr. Herman says. "It comes and goes in varying degrees, but it's always there. The problem with previous formulations of will power is that has been regarded as a trait which is either there or not there, and therefore there's not much you can do about it except develop it through character-building exercises, which probably won't work. Everybody, for instance, is actually capable of resisting food. It's simply a matter of bringing to bear those mental conditions which permit that sort of resistance."

Dr. Herman has studied breakdown of willpower in dieters in three categories:

1. "Binge eating." He found that dieters in his experiments had a threshold of calorie consumption in their minds. If for some reason they went over that threshold, then restraint broke down entirely and they blew their diet. (The test involved feeding enormous milk shakes, followed by ice cream, to dieters and nondieters. Nondieters consumed the milk shakes, then, like any normal animal, managed only a little ice cream. The dieters consumed the milk shakes, then, feeling they had gone over the top, ate very large amounts of ice cream.)

2. Alcohol. Very surprising results emerged from this category. When Dr. Herman gave dieters alcohol *without telling them it was alcohol,* then they kept to their diets. "Alcohol, if you are unaware that it's alcohol you are drinking, seems simply to have a sedative effect on you and makes you feel a little better. And it turns out that feeling better is one of the conditions that helps a dieter stay on her diet. But when we told the subjects it was alcohol they were drinking, then they started losing control and eating more as a consequence." (This says something about alcohol as well as dieting—you need both the alcohol and the perception of it as alcohol in order to get drunk!)

3. Emotional stress. Dr. Herman scared his dieters, and sure enough, they ate more when they were scared than when they were not. The nondieters ate considerably less when they were scared. "Physiologically, the effect of emotional stress ought to be to suppress appetite," he says. "If you are biologically nervous, nature has set things up so that digestion is not what you are particularly concerned with; you are in a 'fight-or-flight' stance which is counterproductive to digestive activity." Dr. Herman thinks that the reason dieters eat more when they are anxious is that for them, self-control or restraint is some kind of mental suppressor of appetite,

and that the emotional stress somehow affects or swamps the restraint mechanism. "If you're worried about something, there's only so much of your mind left over to devote to worrying about staying on your diet."

His newest experiment is probably the most revealing of all. He took his dieters and put them in the same situation as when they had previously overstepped their threshold with the milk shakes, *but with an observer present.* The effect on the dieters was that they rationalized their behavior. They ate just the same, but logically—i.e., eating less when you're full than when you're empty—because they were being watched.

Dr. Herman suggests two important conclusions from this experiment: (1) The dieters could eat perfectly normally when they wanted to, which indicates self-control is there all right, and (2) the presence of an observer made them think, "What would an ordinary person do under these circumstances?" And then they started eating like normal human beings.

What happened was that the dieters became *self-conscious,* and that appears to be one of the keys to self-control.

"Learn to see yourself and what you are doing," says Dr. Herman. "*Self-awareness and self-control are inseparable. You can't have one without the other.*" Ideally we should place an observer in our heads. To some extent we do anyway—we are all social beings, and we carry around other people's opinions of ourselves. (This starts in earliest childhood: "The biggest factor that determines a child's sense of self-esteem is what he thinks his parents think of him," comments psychiatrist Dr. Thomas P. Johnson.)

Self-esteem, the next step in self-awareness, is another aid to self-control. "*People who feel good about themselves feel that they are in control, and remain calm in the face of threats to self-control.*" Dr. James O. Stallings, a plastic surgeon, notes that patients who have had fat removed from their thighs or abdomen by surgery tend not to have problems with overweight again—their self-esteem is so enhanced that they feel good enough about themselves to want to maintain their improved appearance.

The other main path to self-control seems to lie in prevention rather than cure. *"The secret of self-control is anticipation,"* believes Dr. Herman, "learning when you are approaching the boundary of dissipation or lack of control. And you can only learn that through exposure to the experience of going over the top and letting go. Self-exhortation—"Now I'll behave, I'll be good, I promise"—is not an effective method. Experience is really the key, knowing when things are beginning to fall apart." Alcoholics are now being treated with this in mind. Doctors are teaching them to perceive themselves as getting to a danger point *before* it happens, and therefore avoiding disaster.

Another useful thought is to remember that even if you *do* go over the top—eat too much, lose your temper, run from responsibility—it is not going to be the end of the world. All is not lost. "Do not think that once you have passed the threshold you have set for yourself, then all hell breaks loose," advises Dr. Herman. "That way of thinking is very destructive to your self-esteem as well as to your behavior."

There is no doubt that a powerful personal discipline, involving will power or restraint, can help people live more fulfilled lives. There is probably no better example of this than actress Katharine Hepburn, whose long life and career bear witness to her self-determination, rigorous integrity, and indomitable spirit. When asked about codes of conduct, she answered, very simply, "Discipline is totally necessary to the human animal."

How much of this discipline can be inculcated in childhood is not yet known. A study group at Stanford is looking at how children learn to defer their pleasures, and how they develop their capacity to say no to something they want—but very little of the research is conclusive.

For most adults, at any rate, the self-control mechanism is apparently present all the time, and simply functions or not according to the situations we find ourselves in. Dr. Herman thinks that perhaps one day we will be able to call on that elusive mechanism at will, just as people are now understanding enough of how the body works to make physical changes with biofeedback training. "However," he admits, "we are behaviorally, in many respects, far behind our bodies." But that's hardly surprising. After all, what could be more complicated than human behavior?

HOW DO YOU PRACTICE SELF-DISCIPLINE?

It's all very well to know you're supposed to have willpower to control your life—but how do you actually kick it into gear? Here five people, whose professions demand a special kind of self-discipline, tell how they make it work.

Dan Greenburg, humorist and writer, runs two houses, has three cats, and has recently completed a book about his experiences with the occult, *Something's There* (Doubleday).

"I could not possibly handle a free-lance career—or my mortgages—if I were not self-disciplined. I've sort of conned myself into it. The way I do it is this: There are two kinds of activity in my life. One is the physical kind, such as doing errands—getting the typewriter repaired—and the other is creative work. I don't, or can't, do both at the same time. So what I do is kid myself into thinking that when I'm doing the errands I'm getting out of writing, and when I'm writing I'm getting out of the errands.

"Anybody who's successful has to be self-disciplined—but there are extremes. Somebody who's uptight, always keeps a rigid schedule, and won't deviate from it is very boring. But just as boring are the people at the other extreme, who insist on being late for things and going to wild parties even though they aren't having a good time. Hopefully you stay in the middle—lead a relatively structured life, get your work done, and have some fun."

Frank Okamura is a bonsai master at the Brooklyn Botanic

Garden, and teacher of the bonsai-do, the way of the bonsai (growing miniature trees), one of the most intricate and painstaking of all Japanese arts.

"People often ask me, 'Doesn't growing bonsai take a tremendous amount of self-discipline and patience?' My answer is, those words mean you are doing something you do not want to do. Patience means hard work, a hurt heart. Yet the art of bonsai is *enjoying*—understanding what the plant wants. In the West, people seem to want instant results. But the enjoyment of bonsai comes in the feeling of beautiful shapes to come.

"All you must do is study, and continue to study, feeling that one day you will succeed. You must have the feeling, 'I can do it.' If you can hold in your head the dream of what you want to achieve, then you will enjoy the journey toward it."

Martine Van Hamel is a soloist with the American Ballet Theatre, a constant witness to the determination and courage necessary to become a great ballerina.

"Self-discipline is the essence of a dancer's life. All the ingredients of my life go to the idea of perfection—perfection of technique, of musicality, of the body and what it can do. For me, discipline is more than a duty; it becomes a way of life.

"Self-discipline means total concentration on the body—it is that concentration that gets you through. It is like breathing."

Christopher Isherwood has spent a lifetime studying Eastern philosophy, as well as writing such books as *The Berlin Stories, Lions and Shadows,* and more recently, *Christopher and His Kind* (Farrar, Straus & Giroux).

"I'd say I have persistence rather than discipline. It's like fishing rather than gymnastic exercises. There isn't an exactly fixed schedule every day, but some motion of the will is made every day toward writing. It doesn't get any easier, so

I'm not sure that one can learn it. It is an application of the will, and I am very conscious of the struggle.

"But remember it's always easier toward the end; because the opposition, the element of the will that is negative, gives up at a certain point and leaves you free."

Thomas Naegele teaches animation and cartooning at the High School of Art and Design in New York—a profession that surely requires the ultimate in patience and self-control.

"Self-discipline is a basic requirement for a teacher, who must constantly demonstrate how to deal with any and every exigency. I encounter difficult situations in school on occasion, chiefly young people who cannot take responsibilities and act in defiance and provoke exasperation. To avoid a serious confrontation, I try to be polite, firm, positive, and if need be, comical (I have a tendency to be sarcastic, which can backfire badly).

"So many youngsters are merely trying to get attention with their antics. If you snarl or berate them, they will become your enemy—while they really wanted to be your friend."

Chapter 46

HOW TO RELAX

We all know *why* we should relax: to reduce stress, beat high blood pressure, the bane of our fast-paced society, and maintain a healthy heart. But how to do it successfully is sometimes another matter. Today we may feel the need for something more than a good night's sleep to keep a calm frame of mind, and the body and nerves free from knots and tension. Searching for alternate means of relaxation, Dr. Herbert Benson, a Harvard Medical School Professor and cardiologist, and Director, Hypertension Section, Beth Israel Hospital, Boston, and a team of researchers, have investigated mental techniques. And they've discovered some very interesting facts.

Studies show that the human being possesses a *relaxation response*—a mental tool that can be used effectively to soothe and pacify nerves and muscles and generate a comfortable feeling of serenity. In fact, it's a refreshing pause at any time, no matter how you feel! To turn on this relaxation response, all you need to learn is an easy formula for putting your mind to rest:

1

A comfortable position
Sit in a comfortable chair.

2

A quiet environment
Choose a quiet room away from interruptions and noise.

3
A mental device

Turn off everyday thoughts by closing the eyes and focusing either on an object (in the mind's eye), such as a flower, a place, or a person that makes you happy. Or repeat a word you like the sound of over and over.

4
A passive attitude

Discipline yourself to reject ordinary thoughts as they come up by concentrating on the object or word.

5
Regular practice

Do this routine daily—ideally twice a day—for twenty minutes each time.

It all sounds so simple. Why haven't we been doing it before? We have known about it, insists Dr. Benson. "Techniques have existed for centuries for this type of relaxation. There is a repetitive verbal sound in prayer especially in the Catholic religion. And the Jewish religion has a similar type of prayer. In our investigations in the laboratory we have found that such prayers elicit the relaxation response. They take you easily into the meditative state, or an altered state of consciousness. Many of these useful prayers have been neglected."

What actually happens in the meditative state or wakeful rest as it is also called, that produces complete relaxation? Oxygen consumption decreases—"in three or four minutes of meditation you are down to levels that would take four to six hours to reach through sleep," says Dr. Benson—respiratory and heart rates decrease. What these physiological changes add up to is a marked state of decreased sympathetic nervous system activity. In other words, significant bodily relaxation is triggered off through *brain* reaction.

Now there are different methods of mental relaxation

offered by a variety of groups in America today. These methods include Yoga, transcendental meditation (TM), Zen, biofeedback, sentic cycles, self-hypnosis, mind control, Arica, Kundalini. In Dr. Benson's opinion these mental-training groups have all developed a means to a similar end. They are merely offering different ways of training the mind to turn on the relaxation response. If you take up TM—as apparently 450,000 Americans have already done—you may be asked to go to several preliminary lectures, then an initiation ceremony, at which time you pay $120 and obtain a mantra, or word, which is yours personally and is used at home to guide you into the meditative state. A certain mystic quality surrounds TM because of the secrecy of the mantra. However, Dr. Benson concludes that any word repeated over and over will provide the same effect. "Breathe through your nose," he says, "become aware of your breathing. As you breathe out, say the word 'one' silently to yourself. With practice, the relaxation response should come with little effort." If you don't like the word "one," you could substitute "love" or anything else that suits your fancy, adds Dr. Benson. It will have the same result.

Dr. Benson stumbled on mental relaxation first of all by studying hypertension, which causes high blood pressure and heart disease. "We found we could train animals to increase blood pressure and to lower it. While these studies were under way some young people came to me and claimed they, too, had control over their blood pressure and wished to be studied. They practiced TM. I was rather skeptical at first, but at any rate we studied these individuals. Our findings led us to measure other methods of mental relaxation." It is Dr. Benson's conclusion that all these methods of deep, conscious relaxation can only have therapeutic benefit and help us cope with our environment and avoid taking the toll in terms of high blood pressure, strokes, and other hazards.

Apart from feeling more relaxed and less knotted up, people using this mental tool describe other benefits, too— increased clarity of mind, increased productivity in their daily lives. "Many claim to lose their neurotic tendencies and say they are better able to cope, that they decrease their dependency on alcohol, sleeping pills, and other drugs and even cut down on smoking," adds Dr. Benson. "In no way is meditation a substitute for good sleep," he goes on, "but it is a distinct state, which is unique and separate from sleep."

It seems clear that we should all learn to make use of this remarkable asset. As Dr. Benson suggests: Why not take a daily relaxation-response break instead of a coffee break?

Chapter 47

HOW TO USE MORE PERSONAL ENERGY

Solar energy, recycled garbage energy, and many other technological developments are going to change our lives and pull us through the energy emergency. But in the meantime, if we have to push fewer buttons, ride fewer vehicles, this won't be so bad for us, according to Dr. Rene Dubos, eminent microbiologist, environmentalist, pathologist and Professor Emeritus at Rockefeller University. Dr. Dubos believes that if we use more personal energy, we'll very likely live longer, feel better, and enjoy life more.

"Contrary to general belief," declares Dr. Dubos, "longevity has not improved in the last century. Admittedly, statistics show a progressive increase in life expectancy at birth, but this is entirely due to the virtual elimination of child mortality, not to better health or longer survival in adults. There are quite a few centenarians in the world. Their number is less than 10,000 in the United States. In several parts of the world, however, the number is proportionally very much higher than in the U.S. Longevity is often better in countries that are economically poor and where the individual does more himself. The three communities with a high percentage of centenarians have been well documented. They are in the Caucasus highlands of Soviet Georgia, in the

Hunza principality of West Pakistan, and the Andes of Ecuador. The people of these regions are not prosperous and some of them live under conditions that to us are primitive.

"But let's come closer to countries we know better. I'm always startled when I go back to Europe to see people my age—over seventy—or even older out in the countryside and see how active and vigorous they are. All these places have some characteristics in common. Daily caloric intake is extremely low, half that of the average American intake, about 1,200 to 1,800 calories a day, and despite the spartan character of this diet, which seems quantitatively and qualitatively deficient by our standards, the people engage in hard physical work. They are expected to lead an independent life, what's more, an active social role, even when they are past age eighty or one hundred. Throughout their lives they have had to walk and work.

"I'm not preaching or suggesting that we should become more athletic or that there is something fundamentally wrong in using labor-saving machinery, but I think we could all exercise more with beneficial results. You don't have to be an athlete. *The best way to exercise is to do it in the ordinary business of life. You know walking is a wonderfully positive and enriching experience.* It's fun to look at things, see how people dress on the streets, listen to them talk, to feel yourself walk. I'm afraid most people never experience this and are not aware of how much they deprive themselves by not walking. In springtime I walk slowly, trying to feel the softness of the air. If it's fall, I walk briskly and notice everybody looking vigorous. I think those are very small, pleasant experiences of life.

"The American reliance on technology goes extremely deep. We have a habit of substituting indirect experience for direct experience. In my young days, my mother made mayonnaise, beating the oil, the eggs, and all of a sudden the mixture gelled. Now that is a very extraordinary experience. Today you buy mayonnaise in a jar or you make it with a blender, which is very nice and convenient. But you have lost a peculiar pleasure, which comes from something happening because you have done it yourself. If you want to substitute the indirect experience for a direct one, then obviously technological energy helps. You can look at the countryside driving in a car instead of feeling the earth under your feet; if you want to see a snowfall you can turn on the television, instead of actually going out and being in it. Most of the increased standard of living that we talk about has come from providing, without any physical effort, the illusion that you are experiencing the real thing.

"What I'm trying to convey," Dr. Dubos goes on, "is that there are many advantages in our technological society, but that our lives should not be so conditioned that every moment we deprive ourselves of sensations we can have. If you drive through the country and look at nature from inside a car you will lose 90 percent of your ability to smell the air, the grass, and to hear natural noises. Try walking and you will find that at first you start to see general things and you hear vague noises, but within 15 to 20 minutes all of a sudden you begin to be aware of many more things. You hear birds more distinctly, for example. *It's quite extraordinary how the senses can be readily cultivated by putting yourself outside.*

"If you use your eyes, you will develop the ability to perceive. Like anything else, the more you use any part of your body, the more it responds. And this adds to the quality of your life. It makes it so much more interesting. *The development of the sensory experience is the greatest good one can do for people in the world.* But it does take effort to recapture the art of experiencing life directly. I'm not only speaking of sensual or sensory experience, but of total body perception of the world. There is no doubt, you have to be willing to make the initial effort of walking in the snow. Or climbing up a hill. But what an incredible difference, reaching a hilltop by a highway or a funicular and having walked to the top! It's extraordinary, the sensation. It's costly in terms of your effort but it gives you a sense of exhilaration and happiness you would not otherwise experience.

"I stress the need for personal involvement. Well, everybody knows that when a person retires and removes himself completely from life and just sits on the front porch, that this person doesn't last very long. Whereas, if you engage in any kind of activity, I'm not saying that you have to make money or serve the public, but just *do something for which you would like to know the results, this statistically prolongs life.* There is an expectancy for results, a looking forward to the future, which is very important.

"I myself am always planting trees in my garden in the country. Nothing could be more absurd. I'll never see those trees when they're grown; even though I may be as optimistic as I can be, I'm under no illusion about this. But every spring I have an eagerness to see how much my little trees have grown, which makes me very eager to be there next spring, to see whether they have grown a little more. We built a house up in the Hudson River Highlands over twenty years ago. It's isolated and when I think of the social costs, the bringing of electric, telephone, and sewer lines to one place, just for one family, it is extravagant. It's pleasant for us, but socially in many ways, I don't think it's good. The village community where people can gather and talk to each other and walk to shopping places without too much effort is socially a much better way to live. And this allows for an uninterrupted landscape, open space all around, instead of individual houses spotted all over the scenery. Clustering of houses, which many young architects are proposing today, has been done very successfully in places like Vail, Colorado, and I'm sure it will happen progressively all over the land.

"We are going to see much change, change in a most interesting way. Before we had energy as readily available as it has been, people had to design buildings in such a manner that they took advantage of natural conditions. For 5,000

years, architects and people have known and built construc-
tions that were comfortable against heat and cold. I'm almost
sure that in twenty to twenty-five years the individual house
will be powered by local things, sun and wind. And I'm also
sure that using more personal energy will bring a saner,
healthier world and its ultimate result will be a more
creative form of civilization."

THE HOUSE AND GARDEN BOOK
OF
TOTAL HEALTH

RECIPE INDEX

[*] Indicates a low-calorie recipe

THE HOUSE AND GARDEN
BOOK OF
TOTAL HEALTH

INDEX